Heavy Brain

Tommy Caldwell

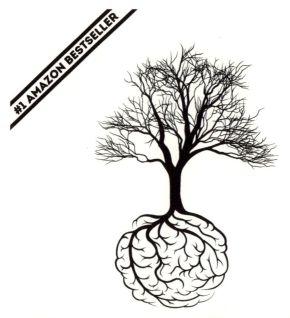

Heavy Brain

HOW TO END LATE NIGHT SNACKING, OVEREATING, AND OTHER BINGE BEHAVIOUR

by Tommy Caldwell

ISBN: 9781983652929

#1 AMAZON BESTSELLER

DEDICATION

This book is dedicated to those who have trusted their health and wellbeing to me over the years. I hope I have served you well and made an impact in your life. I would also like to dedicate this book to my wife, Laura, and my three beautiful children, William, Evelyn, and Madelyn. It is for you that I never stop trying to improve.

ACKNOWLEDGMENTS

I would like to acknowledge my mentors, as well as those individuals who have helped shape the many versions of this book. You know who you are, and I am forever grateful for your time and effort.

MY STORY

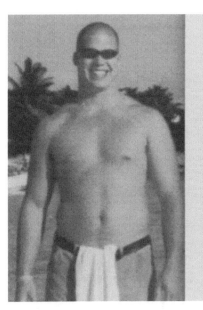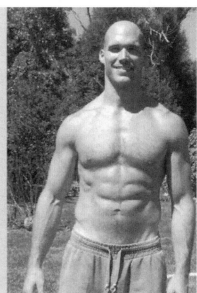

What comes to mind when you see a transformation like the one pictured above? Chances are you assume that I have it all together. I must be one of those lucky people with endless willpower and the discipline of a Buddhist monk. If you saw me hiding under my older sister's bed eating the lifetime supply of chocolate bars she won, day after day, you might change your mind. I finished those chocolate bars in less than two months, before anyone got wise to my gluttony.

When I was a young boy, I was in pain. When my family moved neighbourhoods when I was eight years old, I lost my sense of self. I was bullied, I didn't have any real friends, and I was struggling. I didn't know who I was, and the person I believed myself to be at the time was not a person I liked. I often felt scared, alone, and not good enough. These negative thoughts and feelings pushed me into many unfavourable behaviours. I sacrificed my self in an attempt to fit in, and I lost the ability to be my true self. I sought out a variety of ways to stimulate, numb, and distract myself from the pain I didn't know how to manage. I carried this pain with me through high school and into early adulthood. Even as an athlete, my weight climbed as high as 245 pounds., and I recall eating myself sick, night after night, in an attempt to run from my emotional distress.

This pain, and the attempt to escape it, is what I see in most of my adult clients today. It is the reason why diet and exercise don't work for most people. If you don't understand and solve your motivation for destructive behaviour, it doesn't matter what diet and exercise program you are following. Your fear of failure, negative self-image, and unchecked emotions are going to pull you back to ground zero.

So how did I get to where I am today? How did I become so disciplined and in control of what I put in my body, and of how I move it? It all started in my mind. As soon as I went into the darkness and began to address my psychological motivations for self-destruction, everything changed.

That is what this book is about, and that is the gift I am offering you today. I know what it is like to be in pain. I know what it is like to suffer. I know how it feels to have so little faith in yourself that you are always looking for a way out. Most importantly, I know how to change that mindset and become a success story.

If you know you have a problem inside you that is showing up on your body, and you've had enough, please join me. If you are not yet there, I hope you return in the future.

PREFACE

I didn't write this book because I knew it would sell 100,000 copies. In the world of weight loss, this book isn't the kind that typically sells well. You aren't going to find any tricks or hacks in the pages that follow. The absence of such quick-fix solutions makes for a challenging sales pitch. I could write a book that would sell many copies. I could propose a unique and exciting weight loss approach that seems totally plausible. But if I wrote a book like that, I'd have to sell my soul. Worse, you'd end up with another ineffective weight loss book for your trash can.

Whenever I'm checking out the diet section in my local bookstore, I always see the same themes. How to lose thirty pounds in thirty days. Eat this, not that, and do these exercises. The magic method by celebrity "so and so." I see hundreds of diet books that promise an easy solution to your health and fitness problems. Each comes with a formula that is sold to the reader as unique and compelling. The message of each book is the same: "You have a problem. I have an answer, and the answer is easy and effective." This is the false promise that has made us suckers.

This book does not fit the mold of over-promising and under-delivering. I am going to tell you that the road to long-term weight loss success is not an easy feat. I will tell you that you are likely to 'fail' a few times before you taste sweet victory. I will prove to you that hard work must be done if you are serious about taking back your health. Are you ready to put this book back on the shelf yet?

I'm sure a part of you would prefer the next diet, cleanse, detox, or reset manual instead of a book that talks about the reality of a long, hard, bumpy road. I get it. But you need to ask yourself if any of the tempting "solutions" you have spent thousands of dollars on have worked for you. If you're reading this book, we can assume the quick fixes of the past have not delivered. Whatever you have tried before is clearly not what you needed. This book just might be the thing that works.

At various points while writing this book, I thought to myself, "No one is going to do this much reading to solve their weight loss problem." I hold this view because wanting results in thirty days or less with the least amount of effort is the prevailing mindset. It is the default thinking that props up the multi-billion dollar weight loss industry. At the same time, the overweight and obese populations continue to grow (both literally and figuratively). It doesn't matter that the quick fix solutions we have tried over and over again have never worked for long-term, sustainable weight loss. For some reason, we can't get out of the cycle of spending money on weight loss products that give us hope but not results. The optimist in me believes that people are going to read this book, and something will click. Someone out there wants to resolve their weight problem, and take control of their health, and that person is waiting for a book like this - whether they know it or not. I wrote this book for that person.

The chances are not high that you are the person for whom I wrote this book. Statistically speaking, if you are picking up a book in the hopes that it will solve your weight problems, you are looking to be saved. I hope this is not the case. I want you to be the person who is seeking a reality check by which you can save yourself. If you are hunting for a book that is going to change your life by giving you some sort of magic weight loss solution, you should move on. However, if you are one of the few people willing to forgo the "eat this, not that" approach and focus on deep self-exploration and problem solving, you will succeed.

HOW TO USE THIS BOOK

Before we get to the introductory chapter, I'll tell you how to use this book to get the most out of it. Each chapter will have its main reading content followed by key takeaways and a summary to help clarify how to turn the concepts into action. The summaries are designed to help you apply the content to your life in a meaningful way, and create an internal conversation that highlights your root behavioural problems. Habit and behaviour issues make it impossible to improve your daily choices. Without diving deeply into your behaviours it is very difficult to succeed in your diet and exercise efforts. It is important that we dig these habits and behaviours up early.

When you arrive at any of these sections, I suggest you make notes directly in page margins or on a notepad or your smartphone. Where you decide to document your personal work is up to you. I would just encourage you to do the work. If it feels tedious, you can skip it and come back to it later, or forego the note making. In the coming pages I have written descriptions of what each section contains, as well as what you will find in each chapter. You can read the book from start to finish (which is what I suggest), or skip directly to sections that sound most relevant to your needs. There isn't a right or wrong way to read the book. Just be sure to intimately understand the core concepts and how they relate to your life. Make this book work for you.

INTRODUCTION

I have spent more than half my life working in the health and fitness industry, and I must admit that I despise what it has come to represent. Perhaps this stems from millions of "coaches" and "personal trainers" that I have been exposed to since the rise of Instagram. These are people whose main qualifying factor for a fitness job is the shape of her butt or the size of his biceps. In any case, I have developed a strong distaste for what the health and fitness industry has come to represent. Not to mention the fact that statistically speaking, we aren't helping anyone.

Obesity rates and lifestyle-based diseases are skyrocketing. People are getting fatter and sicker with every passing year. If the number of people who died each year from obesity-driven diseases were dying from a virus, bug bites, or terrorism, we'd all demand an immediate solution. You can spin the reality of our health however you like. Still, the fact is that whatever the health and fitness industry is offering the world, it is not working for more than 95% of the population. Of all the North Americans who attempt to get to a healthy body weight, less than 1 in 20 will find long-term success. This dismal outcome is in spite of billions of dollars spent on weight loss solutions like diet books, gym memberships, online programs, pills, powders, and home fitness.

Fitness professionals believe that we are actively improving the health of our clients. Still, when you look at the actual statistics, there isn't any reason to believe that. I couldn't imagine the general public using any other service that failed to deliver on its intended result less than 5% of the time. Statistically speaking, we all suck at what we do. What qualifies a person as a fitness professional, anyway?

This is the first question worth asking. It seems that as long as you have revealing clothing in your closet, filters on your smartphone, and a semi-popular social media account, you qualify to lead others. However, it requires a well-trained eye to spot an educated professional through the fog of Instagram butt models and multi-level marketing snake oil salespeople. I can only speak for myself when I say I have become embarrassed to have the word 'fitness' or 'coach' next to my name. Those words have become meaningless.

The world of health, fitness, and weight loss is dishonest, ineffective, costly, arrogant, superficial, and, worst of all, ignorant of these facts. The "unknown unknowns" that Donald Rumsfeld warned us about could not be stronger and more prevalent than in fitness professionals. There are great coaches out there who are doing their best to help people, but they are in the minority. The fitness industry is failing, yet everyone continues to operate as if we are being effective.

Slapping the face of an industry that I have spent 20 years of my life working in is not going to win me any popularity contests. I am not concerned with the attitudes of my peers. I don't respect or care for most of these people because I see them as frauds. I'm sure they are all beautiful people in some way, but many are doing a lousy job and simply don't care. I can't be concerned with backlash. If I want to write this book the way it needs to be written to make an impact, I need to be brutally honest.

If I can't get you to change the way you think about your health, I have to question the point of my professional existence. I have coached thousands of people, including some of the world's elite athletes. I have opened multiple gyms that have housed enthusiastic members and the best coaching staff you'll find under one roof. I have consulted for sports teams and rewarding community organizations.

That is all well and good, but I have yet to make a dent in the mountain-sized issue of weight gain, obesity, and preventable disease. This is the only problem worth solving.

Heavy Brain will challenge everything you think you know about diet and exercise. That will be difficult for you because you have spent your life believing that diet and exercise is the key to your weight loss success.

I hope you are open to new possibilities. It will be natural to resist the truth, and there are a few reasons why it will be difficult for you to move past diet and exercise centricity. Here are a few of those reasons.

1.   Every T.V. doctor, personal trainer, and nutritionist on the face of the planet has touted diet and exercise strategies as the key to health and longevity. Eat this, not that, and you will get everything you want out of your body. This is a lie you have been repeatedly told, and everyone is in on it.

2.   What you eat and how you move are easy concepts to understand, which makes them appealing to apply. You already have a framework for what diet and exercise are and how each works. They are familiar to you, and you are comfortable with them. Diet and exercise can also provide you with quick feedback. "If I am sweating, this must be working!" Immediate feedback biases us to believe the activity is more worthwhile.

3.   The long-term solution to your health problems requires that you face your own issues. You need to own up to your weaknesses, dismantle your excuses, and put a significant amount of work into your well-being. That task is a lot harder than eating celery, running on a treadmill, or

taking a pill. The necessary work is often avoided because it is complicated and scary. Results come slowly, and the process is a bit of a rollercoaster. Most people would rather just be overweight than face any of that.

You'll need to overcome these lies and biases if you want to succeed. Otherwise, you will spend your life searching for progress in all the wrong places without actually getting anywhere.

Sections

This book has three parts, each with its own purpose.

Part 1: The Barriers to Success (and how to overcome them)

The first section of the book addresses our beliefs about success and failure in fitness. This section will explain why your current beliefs are false and how these beliefs are preventing you from reaching your goals. This will help you to identify the deep psychological issues that lead to failure in fitness. The barriers to success are the primal paradox, our toxic culture, laziness, and the need to self-medicate with food, alcohol, and technological distraction. Overcoming the barriers may sound complicated, and it is. Still, once you appreciate the information in this section, it will all make sense. You will be empowered and perhaps even enlightened - both awakenings you need to move toward long-term solutions. You will become well versed in how our evolutionary faults, adverse life experiences, societal pressures, and unhelpful brain play a role in the struggle to be healthy. You will identify your unique "isms" that lead you to overeat, snack when you aren't hungry, be lazy and distracted, and store a lot of fat. You will also learn how the adverse life events you've experienced influence the food you put in your mouth today.

By the end of Part 1, you will understand the problems that prevent you from succeeding. This includes how they play out in your life, and what you can do to change your most unhealthy, self-sabotaging behaviours.

Part 2: Preparing Yourself for Change

In the second section of the book, I will show you how to lay the groundwork for success. This will help you to implement practical solutions to the problems you will identify in Part 1. Humans have a tendency to harness fleeting moments of inspiration and jump into diet and exercise programs without a real plan. We try sophisticated strategies before we are actually in a position to help ourselves, which leads to a high rate of failure. We don't lay any of the groundwork needed to create a foundation for success. This lack of preparation and rush for results leaves us open to the self-sabotaging thoughts, feelings, and actions that result in failure. Ego protecting systems and various forms of denial destroy us before we reach our goal. This is the number one reason why most of us repeatedly fail and never find success and happiness in our personal health. By the end of Part 2, you will understand why you always seem to be your own worst enemy, and what you can do to start being an ally for your health instead.

Part 3: Taking Your Mind (and Body) Back

All of the sections in this book are critical for your long-term success, but Part 3 is where you will find most of the strategies. At this point in the book, you will understand why the keys to weight loss, improved health, and long-term results begin in your mind. I will teach you how you can create an operating system that leads you towards your goals. I will show you how to change your most unhealthy behaviours, so you can stick to your diet and exercise efforts once and for all. We will also touch on lifestyle factors like sleep quality and stress management that must be addressed to support your behavioural change.

By the end of Part 3, you will know how to access the power of your mind and reach your goals. You will also learn the supporting lifestyle exercises you can introduce to help reinforce your success.

By the end of the book

When you complete this book, you will possess the tools required to take control of your health. You will understand what is preventing you from succeeding and how you can overcome those barriers. You will learn to see yourself in a light that leads to positive outcomes and an increase in healthy behaviours. You will learn how to prevent self-sabotage and bypass the default operating system that is currently controlling your fate. In short, you will have everything you need to finally take advantage of diet and exercise strategies, overcome failure, and get results.

Chapter Breakdown

The 3 sections of this book contain the following chapters I believe you will get the most out of the book by reading it start to finish, but perhaps that won't work for you. I am listing the basics of what each chapter has to offer so you can focus on sections that might give you immediate benefits. Feel free to jump around and read ahead if that is what you prefer to do.

Chapter 1: The Lies We Believe About Weight Loss
Before you can get to a solution, you need to identify the problem. Most of us do not understand the problem. Therefore we fall for sterile solutions. That is what we will discuss here. In this chapter, I cover the false realities of weight loss. I detail why our shared beliefs are problematic and reveal the truth behind what is driving our health difficulties. This information is critical for those who get stuck in cycles of failure.

Chapter 2A: The Primal Paradox
We are designed to fail. If you don't understand this, you will beat yourself up unnecessarily. I wrote this chapter so you can understand why it is so difficult to make healthy choices even when you are motivated to make a change. Your current state of health isn't your fault, but it is your responsibility. Understanding the primal roots of unhealthy human behaviour can aid you in this process.

Chapter 2B: Our Toxic Culture
The modern society is one of abundance. We have millions of calories of hyper-palatable food within a one block radius at all times. We can be constantly distracted with thousands of hours of media at our fingertips. We are also part of a growing digital pseudo-society filled with fake

Instagram lives and constant social pressures. It as if the world around us has been built to play into our deeply ingrained primal maladaptations.

Chapter 3: How Adverse Life Experiences Drive Self-Medication

Adverse life experiences, modern stress, and a culture that makes us feel "small" hurt our health. In this section, I will shine the light on what drives us to overeat, stare at the T.V., and take part in many behaviours that act as a form of self-medication. Knowing what these common pathways look like and where they are coming up in your life is an essential step toward taking control of your most harmful habits. Emotional suffering is the common cause of our most unhealthy habits. Learn where you are self-medicating and why.

Chapter 4: The Unhealthy Reward Cycle

Chapters 1-3 are introductions to a complex problem. In this chapter, I show the reader how these barriers come up in "real life." How does the combination of our old brain and modern environment turn into unrelenting cravings, overeating, technological addiction, and laziness? How do emotions and underlying stresses contribute to unhealthy decision-making? Real-world examples will be found here.

Chapter 5: Are you Ready to Change?

Many of us attempt to take control of our health before we are ready to take meaningful action. In this chapter, I will teach you how to assess your readiness and build the fundamentals for success. If you have not created a strong foundation for behaviour change, motivation becomes meaningless. I will teach you how to identify the areas where you are exposing yourself to failure and where you might need to do some work before you transform your health.

Chapter 6: The Myth of Motivation
Our success is obsessively measured by metric-based goals like the number on the scale. It is a better long-term strategy to be driven by daily actions that you can use to measure your progress. Our relationship with our bodies causes needless anxiety and prevents a strong relationship with our "self." This section will teach you how to set better goals for yourself and to measure those goals positively.

Chapter 7: The Lifestyle Levers of Success
20% of your efforts are responsible for 80% of your results. In my experience, this is true. Most of us overlook the small impactful actions we can take while obsessing over the useless ones. We desperately try to figure out the perfect fat burning heartrate while only sleeping four hours per night or seek out magic weight loss pills while stress eating into a food coma. In this chapter, I will discuss why undervalued levers like sleep quality and stress management are so crucial for long term success, and how you can begin to improve these underutilized areas of your health for maximal results.

Chapter 8: Training Your Brain for Change
Exercising your mind is a non-negotiable action for long-term success. It is the area where we are most weak, but the area where we give the least effort. Before, during, and after our most unhealthy actions, there are opportunities to reinforce better decision-making. And decision-making ability is what makes the difference between success and

failure. In this chapter, I will teach you how to implement this process and break your most challenging, unhealthy habits.

Chapter 9: In the Event of a Relapse...
Success does not operate in a straight line. You know this, but you rarely accept the weight-loss rollercoaster ride. You will fall off the wagon. You will relapse. Even after a year of great success, you will be open to slip-ups. Heck, I've personally had bad weeks, months, seasons, and years! The more committed you are to your success, the more relapses you will face. As long as you know how to recognize regressions when they surface and understand what actions you can take, the situation can be a real growth opportunity. In this chapter, I will teach you what to do in such cases so you can turn the process of relapse into a chance to grow and become even more successful.

CHAPTER 1-THE LIES WE BELIEVE ABOUT WEIGHT LOSS

"It isn't that they cannot find the solution. It is that they cannot see the problem." – **G.K Chesterton**

I want to begin the opening chapter of this book by telling you a few stories that will help you understand what we believe to be true about weight loss. These are the beliefs that the vast majority of the fitness world pushes onto clients and customers daily, theories that have collectively produced a dismal 5% industry success rate.

The problem with false beliefs is that they prevent you from understanding the truth you must grasp to find success. There are real barriers that are preventing you from implementing solutions that work. As long as you continue to hang onto false beliefs about the source of your struggles, you will continue to search for answers in the wrong places. If you believe that you have a flat tire because there isn't enough air in it, you put air in the tire. But what if the tire is actually punctured? You will repeatedly fill that tire with air, always resulting in another flat within a few hours. You would wake up scratching your head and wondering why air keeps disappearing from your perfectly adequate tire. If you understood, however, that the underlying issue was due to a hole, you could just patch

1

it and solve the problem. False beliefs in fitness work the same way. We fill the fitness tire up with gadgets, trendy exercise programs, online weight loss products, and supplements. Then we wonder why we never get anywhere.

Less than 1 in 20 people succeed with "help" from the weight loss industry, and this lack of achievement is due to inaccurate industry-wide beliefs. So why don't fitness professionals smarten up and change the approach to be more productive? What is the point in continuing with strategies that obviously aren't working for people? I will answer these later on in the book. For now, I will just say that the combination of ego and bias is preventing professionals from being objective and self-critical enough to be useful. It is clear that we are not helping anyone, but it is too painful for the industry to shift gears. If you dedicate your life to a specific strategy, it would be natural to focus on the few successes you achieve while ignoring your failures. This would be especially true if your livelihood and financial stability depended on people believing that you have a solution for their problem. This is what is happening in the health, fitness, and weight loss world today. Look at any weight loss company's promoted success stories. What you are seeing in "before and after" pictures is one person out of twenty who got a result. The 19 other failures are, of course, not mentioned. Commonly promoted weight loss success stories are also just snapshots that don't equate to a long-term result. The accomplishment only has to exist long enough to have before and after pictures taken.

If you don't know much about the ego, biases, and heuristics that prevent professionals from ditching their failing systems, we will be covering these in the book. For the time being, we need to establish the false beliefs that prevent us from getting to the source of our fitness failures.

If you understand these common erroneous beliefs, you can begin to move toward the solution. Here are a few stories that I hope will help you see yourself in the following false beliefs.

Note: I will summarize the purpose of all three stories at the end of the third story.

Brenda and Eric

Brenda is aging. She isn't old by any means, but she is no longer in the mid to late twenty-something range that most would consider being "young." She looks at herself in the mirror each morning and feels as though she can see herself aging. She is in her mid-thirties and becoming increasingly concerned about her weight and physical appearance.

Brenda put on a few pounds back in university. This sort of thing is typical of that time in the life of both young men and women - and she added a few more pounds to her frame in her early professional years. By the time of her 34th birthday, Brenda weighed 50pounds more than she did in high school. Gulp.

It goes without saying that these days, Brenda does not like what she sees in the mirror. She is also suffering many of the other everyday reminders of her slipping health. For instance, when she recently tried on a pair of pants that were purchased just 6 months ago, she could no longer do up the zipper. Despite many attempts to contort and 'will' her way into the pants, the result was the same. She couldn't fathom that her body would be growing at this rate. These sorts of cumulative reminders of Brenda's slipping health have left her psychologically destroyed and in an unhealthy emotional state.

Eric is a young personal trainer and nutritionist at a

reasonably reputable gym that is close to Brenda's work. He is enthusiastic about his job, and he cares about his clients. He is considered to be one of the few excellent local trainers. A few of Brenda's colleagues have attended Eric's group weight loss classes and speak very highly of him. He's also not hard on the eyes, which seems to be an additional selling point - even if just for the visual distraction from the pain of exercise. One of the women in the group suggests that Brenda set up a consult with Eric to discuss a customized fitness and nutrition plan that Brenda can do on her own. Something structured and straightforward that Brenda can reference and follow to get her health (and her confidence) back. Brenda takes the suggestion.

A week later, Brenda finds herself sitting in Eric's small, but professional looking office. There's a scale, some measuring tapes, body fat calipers, and the classic picture of a cat hanging desperately from a tree branch with the underlying quotation, 'hang in there'! Brenda isn't sure if the cat picture is to be taken seriously or if it is supposed to be satirical, but nonetheless, it makes her smile. Eric enters the room, and they begin with a greeting and some typical small talk before getting right into the heart of the matter. Eric wants to know how much weight Brenda would like to lose and how much time she would like to have lost that amount of weight. He asks what she currently does for exercise, as well as some general questions about her daily diet. He asks all of the questions you would expect to be asked considering what Brenda is there for. It appears that Eric is collecting all of the correct information. Brenda explains that she would like to lose 50 pounds. "ASAP" and get her high school body back. Eric is familiar with this common "want" and begins his diagnostics. Eric takes Brenda's girth measurements, calculates her body fat, measures her scale weight and height, and performs all of the other "how fat are you" metrics.

Brenda waits patiently (or perhaps anxiously) while Eric performs some calculations. "Well, Brenda," Eric says, "your body fat is currently at 39%, and your BMI is in the mid-thirties. You have a lot of weight to lose." Tell Brenda something she doesn't know. "But the good news is that I can help you," Eric says. "It will take hard work and dedication on your part, but if you just do what I ask of you and do your best every day, we will get you to your goal!" Brenda is naturally skeptical of Eric's promise to turn her weight gain around but becomes hopeful and intrigued by his confidence in the matter.

Eric tells Brenda that he is going to send her a diet plan and an at-home exercise program within the next three days. He suggests that she should begin following them both immediately. Every month she is to come into his office for a "weigh-in" so he can check her progress and make any necessary changes to the program. The instructions have been laid out, the program is in Brenda's possession, and it is time to see how this thing goes.

Without hesitation, Brenda gets started on her new program. She hits the grocery store with Eric's custom shopping list. She aggressively cleans the junk food out of her cupboards, begins preparing meals and snacks for the coming workweek, and begins her at-home workouts. Brenda is inspired and jumping into her program with both feet. She is motivated, she is determined, and she is already feeling satisfaction just from the act of getting started. Brenda feels great!

A few weeks go by, and everything is looking good. Brenda is down 10 pounds. and feeling confident. The initial weight loss is likely from the decreased water retention that is expected from the lowered carbohydrate intake that Eric suggested, but who cares, 10 pounds. are something to celebrate! Eric's system is delivering results, and Brenda could not be happier.

At Brenda's first check-in, she has lost 3% body fat and is sent home with a "prescription" to continue doing what she has been doing. Why change anything when the process is working? Eric is happy, Brenda is ecstatic, and they both have adequate fuel for a little "back-patting." But as it usually goes in the early phases of weight loss, the enthusiasm does not last as long as Brenda hoped it would.

Over the next month, things don't appear to be going quite so well for Brenda. As the weeks go by, her progress rapidly slows down. In fact, it has completely stopped. Nothing has changed for Brenda. She is still doing her best to watch what she eats and stay active. She continues to follow all the steps that Eric has suggested, but she isn't losing any more weight. Worse than that, it appears that she may even be gaining back some of the weight from her initial 10-pound loss. Brenda goes into full-on panic mode and schedules an emergency check-in with Eric.

At the check-in, the results aren't as positive as they were the first time around. This is no surprise given the lack of progress that has led to Brenda's current "meltdown." Brenda is up 3 pounds. since her last check-in, and her body fat measurement is almost the same as at her initial meeting with Eric. The fat that she lost has returned, and it seems as though all the progress that was motivating Brenda just a few weeks ago has now been undone. Eric asks a series of questions relating to Brenda's diet and exercise regimen to investigate what has happened. Has Brenda really been exercising the way she claims to have been? Is Brenda really following the dietary advice that Eric had laid out for her? Has Brenda really been following this plan at all? Eric suggests that Brenda eat less food and increase her activity level, thus increasing her "caloric deficit." This is a classic move for increasing progress on the scale. This is a strategy that many of us intrinsically implement when we don't like the amount of stomach fat we can grab while sitting at the breakfast table. We increase our time on the treadmill and become highly restrictive with our food intake. This is our first line of defence against body fat.

Eric follows this industry trend and prints off a new food plan with a further reduction in carbohydrates and overall calories. He also adds in an extra exercise session per week for Brenda to fit into her schedule. Brenda accepts the new plan and walks out the door feeling a little defeated and considerably less hopeful than she felt after the last meeting. This doesn't mean she is going to quit. Still, her once motivated mind is now becoming filled with familiar negative self-talk. The voice says, "You're not good enough to take control of your health. You're too weak and undisciplined. This is why you're fat and why you'll never be fit again." It's a nasty little voice that becomes the prominent source of conversation in Brenda's mind. It's the kind of sound that is quite familiar to most of us.

In spite of her emotional stress, Brenda starts over and follows the new instructions laid out by Eric. She shops for a bit less food and throws out much of what is in her cupboards. She adds in the extra exercise session each week. After week one of the updated plan, Brenda is hungry, lethargic, and a bit foggy in the brain. This is probably due to the drop in calories and increase in exercise. Combine those with the stress, frustration, and sadness that are building in her mind. Brenda soldiers on. Another week goes by, and Brenda is now just desperately hanging on. Days go by, and she has little to no energy, she is becoming increasingly depressed, and all she can think about is food. Brenda has a brief mental snapshot of the "hang in there" poster in Eric's office with the cat hanging from the tree branch. Brenda is no cat, she thinks. By the end of the week, Brenda is so low in energy and so ravenously hungry that she can no longer stand it. Brenda breaks down and begins eating through every piece of food in the house. She goes to the fridge, the pantry, and the freezer. Brenda eats cookies, crackers, cheese, and chocolate. She can't stop. Her brain has picked up on the rapid stimulation of incoming calories and relentlessly begs for more. The more Brenda eats, the harder it becomes to stop eating. She gets to the point where she doesn't even taste the food anymore, and her food mannerisms are similar to those seen at hot dog eating contests. The level of consumption is impressive.

Flash forward to an hour later. Brenda is lying on the couch and watching T.V. She has slumped into a food-driven depression. Her stomach hurts, her mouth is sore and dry from all the salty snacks and sugar Brenda consumed, and a food hangover is beginning to set in. She is ashamed of herself. She feels a sensation of overwhelming guilt, and the voice in her head has returned for the final blow. "Here you are, Brenda. Doing precisely what we all knew Brenda would do. Your transformation journey is over. Welcome back to your real life and the real you."Defeated, sad, and destroyed, Brenda has officially quit her fitness plan.

Susan and John

Susan is your average, everyday, middle-aged woman. Forty-nine to be exact. With every passing year, Susan becomes increasingly concerned with her expanding waistline and the hormonal cascade that looms over most women like a dark cloud: menopause.

Over the last five years, Susan has tried every trick, method, gadget, and supplement available in an attempt to take control of her health. If you can name it, it is sitting in her basement. Workout DVD's, ab wheels, belly shockers, and discarded weight-loss shake containers that were going to be the next big fat-burning machine litter her closets and garage. The list of purchases made by Susan in desperate attempts to lose weight is in the tens of thousands of dollars. You almost have to admire Susan's commitment to purchasing her way out of her health problems.

All in all, Susan has spent nearly $20,000 over the last 5 years on these "quick fix" solutions and hasn't lost a single pound, at least not a pound that she has been able to keep off. Even worse than that, year after year, she is continuing to gain weight.

In spite of the evidence that the quick-fixes she has purchased have not resulted in any long term weight-loss, Susan continues to believe that the right product is out there. She tells herself that perhaps she just has not found it yet. This mentality is at its peak when Susan is up at 2 AM, feeling particularly bad about herself, and with her eyes glued to the latest fat-burning machines on the shopping network.

Aware of Susan's ongoing health frustrations, a friend tells her about an online weight loss program. The friends (let's call her Jane) claims that this program has changed her life. You see, Jane used to be in the same situation as Susan. Jane was once growing increasingly heavy, scared of lifestyle-based diseases, and frustrated with her state of health. But these days Jane looks slim, secure, and happy.

Like most people who have seen recent success in weight loss, Jane is now an evangelist for her online program and her weight loss coach, John. The structure and accountability of the program that comes with having her own personal coach have seemingly worked wonders for Jane. Therefore in Jane's mind, everyone should use the program and coach that got her results.

The online program and coach that Jane swears by aren't cheap. Still, if they can deliver the results that Susan has been desperately striving after for all these years, the cost is irrelevant. At the encouragement of her friend, Susan decides to take her suggestions and contact the magical online personal trainer, John.

Flash-forward to a month later, and Susan has officially become a client of John's online weight loss program. For the past few weeks, Jane has been speaking to John once per week through Skype to go over diet, exercise, and lifestyle interventions. So far, so good. John is both knowledgeable and motivating, and Susan likes the structure, accountability, and encouragement that comes with the online program. Susan has dropped 6 pounds in just 2 weeks, and although she wishes she were down closer to 10 pounds, she is happy.

John has Susan on a strict eating plan, he holds her accountable to her exercise routine, and it all seems to be working for the two of them. Although the program is just in the very early phases, Susan is happy and hopeful of where it will take her.

Another month goes by, and things aren't going quite as well as they did in the first month. Susan is still talking to John once per week and doing her best with her diet and exercise program. The scale, however, is not showing any further progress.

Susan feels stuck, frustrated, and confused. Underneath that sense of confusion is the same little voice that haunted Brenda. The same underlying internal messages are being sent to Susan as well. Thoughts like, "Here we go. It was only a matter of time. You knew that this process wouldn't work for you. You're hopeless and should just give up," begin to plague Susan's mind. She is digging herself into a ditch of failure mentality, a place known all too well by most dieters.

John and Susan decide to get on a call to discuss her current lack of progress and what can be done to restart it. John asks Susan a variety of in-depth questions about her diet and where she may be slipping up. Susan admits to snacking late at night when she is bored. Susan has also been missing breakfast when she is rushed, eating out quite a bit, and often going an entire day without thinking about her food choices. Susan is only human, right?

John decides that it is time to increase Susan's level of activity and further restrict her diet. John is authoritative in reminding Susan that, "If she cared about losing weight, she would cut out the unhealthy actions that aren't on his 'approved' list." A little shaming goes a long way in John's mind, and that is the only way to make more progress, he tells Susan. John and Susan are both anxious to make up for what seems like lost time in her transformation journey.

The two exit the phone call with silent thoughts about Susan's current lack of progress. John believes that Susan isn't losing weight because she is not committed and doesn't value her health the way she says she does. If she actually cared, she would do what he asked, every day, without fail. No excuses. Since she has had some dietary slip-ups in the last month, he can only conclude that she lacks commitment and willpower. John does not verbalize his thoughts and feelings to Susan, and he has already mentally moved beyond the possibility of Susan's success. He has seen her type before, and she simply doesn't have "what it takes."

Susan walks away with destructive feelings that have been internalized. Susan sees herself as weak, stupid, and undeserving of the healthy changes that she wants so badly. The way Susan subconsciously feels about herself on most days is rising to the surface of her mind and becoming more prominent in her thinking. Why else would she have so much trouble sticking to a restricted dietary structure? Susan says to herself, "This is why I am fat. Because I am a weak, uncommitted loser who doesn't deserve to be happy and healthy." The awful little voice that underlies most of our thoughts and feelings has taken hold of Susan and is now in control.

It is only a matter of time until Susan begins missing weekly calls with John and slipping back into her old ways. John is expecting this 'relapse' from Susan. He is already telling himself that he will no longer have to waste his time with a person who clearly doesn't care about her health. John is content to collect his remaining paycheque and move onto more ambitious clients. Susan, on the other hand, will be destroyed. She will fall into a dark place of shame and low self-worth for some time. Then she will go back to desperately seeking the magic pill, technology, or piece of exercise equipment that will change her life. This is the cycle of failure that Susan (and many like Susan) are stuck in.

Ryan and Maggie

Ryan and Maggie have never known what it feels like to be 'skinny.' Since the day they first met (almost seven years ago), they have only known themselves to be a heavy-set couple. Despite their best efforts to lose weight, they have never made any progress that lasted for more than a few months.

Ryan and Maggie, while raised individually with their own family experiences, had very similar upbringings. Food was a big part of their lives, and you'd be hard-pressed to find a close relative of either who wasn't also struggling with his or her weight.

Candy and treats were available around the clock for the pair from a very young age. Food was often used to keep Maggie quiet when she was "acting up" or to reward Ryan for what his parents deemed to be ideal behaviour. Participation in formal exercise or community sports was never a significant concern for either of their families. Ryan and Maggie have both been "big" for as long as they can remember, and each came from families made up of other "big" people, who took part in all of the unhealthy lifestyle behaviours that you would associate with obese families.

Regardless of having the fitness cards stacked against them, Ryan and Maggie have tried countless interventions to turn their health around. They have been in and out of weight watchers enough times to count on two hands. They have a shelf full of dusty old diet books and a closet packed with exercise gadgets. But none of these modalities has resulted in long-term health outcomes for the young couple. This lack of results has never been for a lack of desire to improve their health. For some reason, the pair just cannot seem to make any of their efforts produce results and "stick."

In a last-ditch effort, Ryan and Maggie decided to join a couple's weight loss retreat in Mexico that came across Maggie's Facebook feed. Ten days of cleansing, organic foods, enemas, and exercise will round out the retreat agenda. Most of that sounds pretty great to Ryan and Maggie, except for the obvious (the saline solution being shot up their butts). On an isolated retreat, there wouldn't be anywhere to go for junk food, nor would there be any escape from the daily regime of health interventions provided by the resort staff. Ryan and Maggie would not have any way to sabotage the health intervention, and if this wouldn't work for them, nothing would.

Ryan and Maggie committed to the retreat and spent ten wonderful, yet trying, days away in the name of a personal health revolution. The rigorous schedule of exercise, juice only "meals", and the routine shooting of water into their colons seem to have done something. After the 10 day journey, both Ryan and Maggie each lost over twenty pounds. Twenty pounds in ten days. Not bad. In fact, after the adjustment period in the first few days, they had actually started to enjoy the routine.

Ryan and Maggie felt as if they were in control. "There is hope," they thought.

The pair walked away from the retreat feeling motivated and ready to take their health into their own hands. They might not be able to keep up with everything they experienced at the retreat, but most of what they learned while away could be maintained in their day-to-day lives.

Upon returning home, Ryan and Maggie were inspired to stick to the diet and exercise continuation plan provided to all of the retreat guests by the resort staff. This at-home routine included an emphasis on fresh fruit and vegetables, low to no animal protein, healthy fats, and lots and lots of juicing. Ryan and Maggie committed themselves to what they started on the retreat, and they did a great job of keeping each other accountable to the structure they were to follow.

A few weeks passed, and as per the home program, it was time to step back onto the scale and see how much further the pair had come. Ryan and Maggie held each other's hand (and their breath) as they nervously transferred their weight onto their respective bathroom scales. Ryan and Maggie looked down with shock. Paralyzing disappointment hit the pair. The scale revealed that they had each gained back almost 1/2 of what they had lost during the retreat. "How is this possible?" they thought. "We have stuck to everything that was asked of us for the last 2 weeks, and we've each gained back 50% of the weight we lost?!" Unable to hold back her emotions, Maggie broke down crying. Ryan did his best to stay strong and comfort his sobbing wife, but what he felt on the inside was precisely what Maggie was expressing on the outside. Hope turned to pain. Motivation turned to disappointment. Ryan and Maggie were shattered.

Just like our other weight loss industry victims, Ryan and Maggie begin to internalize negativity. This must be about their character. This must be a matter of uncontrollable flaws. The harsh automatic thoughts that stem from their underlying belief systems begin to rage and take over. This reinforced the belief that they were born fat, they grew up fat, and they will die fat, likely at a much younger age than the average person. "You're fat, you're useless, you're disgusting, you'll never be normal." These are the kinds of thoughts that begin to run through Ryan's and Maggie's minds.

After a few challenging and emotional hours, the couple does their best to gather their collective selves and sit down to ask, "What now?" They spend the following hour looking for whom or what they can blame for their seemingly impossible weight circumstances. They have done everything possible to lose weight and be healthy. They have followed the advice of physicians, personal trainers, nutritionists, and celebrity gurus. They have tried. They really have. What else can the pair possibly do?

After much rumination, the two are left with only one logical conclusion. It must be their genetics. What else could be dooming them to a life of obesity in the face of all the efforts? This must be the result of some genetic curse that sealed the fate of their weight long ago. It is a convenient hypothesis for the two that gives an answer while also removing responsibility and blame. A little bit of Googling and Ryan managed to find some interesting literature about "fat" genes and "laziness" genes that might explain their personal obesity hypothesis.

"We are fat because our parents are fat, and we will die fat just like our grandparents died." In the minds of Ryan and Maggie, they never stood a chance. Any efforts they made in the past to improve their weight had been rendered ineffective by their genetic predispositions. Ryan has even found the "science" to back it.

So what do the two conclude? They might as well go back to doing the things that make them happy: overeating, late-night snacking, hours of T.V. every night, and copious amounts of social eating and drinking. "If we are going to die young and fat," they think, "we might as well do it on our own terms!" An all too familiar scenario.

The purpose of the three stories

So what was the point of telling these three stories to kick off the book? What am I trying to illustrate here?

When you are trying to solve a problem in your life (in this case, a weight or health problem), the first step you must take is understanding what the problem is and is not. Many times we believe solutions begin with identifying only what the problem is, but we rarely get that part of the equation correct. We rarely identify the core issues that are leading to our adverse health outcomes.

This inability to identify our core issues stems from a misunderstanding of the problem. Like the great Charles

Kettering said, "a problem well stated is a problem half-solved." Unfortunately, like the people and professionals seen in the three storytelling examples, we are usually stating the wrong set of problems, and thus we implement the wrong set of solutions.

The stories you just read demonstrate some of the most common misunderstandings or myths in the world of weight loss. I formulated them in the way that they usually play out in our own lives. Chances are that if you have a weight problem, you saw yourself in one or all of those stories. And chances are that it was uncomfortable to read some of those examples. If so, that is a good sign. It means that this book is likely going to help you.

There are likely countless myths you currently believe about weight loss and your body. Myths that are preventing you from taking control of your health. I am going to bring to your attention the three that I see most frequently in my coaching business.

The 3 Weight Loss Myths

Perhaps you gained a real sense of the 3 myths by reading the stories I presented to you. They are somewhat obvious, but that is easy for me to say since I already know what they are. Assuming you didn't catch them, let me state them here. The 3 biggest myths in weight loss that we are told (and believe) that prevent us from identifying the actual problem(s) are that:

1. **Diet and exercise are the keys to weight loss**
2. **When we can't stick to diet and exercise plans, it is because we are weak and uncommitted**
3. **If we make our best diet and exercise efforts and do not succeed it is due to genetic predispositions**

Does any of this sound familiar? Let me explain in detail why each one of these beliefs is 100% false (at least in the way they are taught to us and in the way in which we understand them to be true). It should also be noted that if you cannot see these beliefs as false, you will never succeed. That isn't just me trying to encourage you to believe what I have to say. It is only the reality of the situation. If you continue thinking that diet and exercise efforts are the keys to weight loss, that your lack of commitment is a character flaw, and that the source of your health issue is genetic, you will continue to get sucked into an unhelpful mindset. This is an inaccurate set of stated problems that push you into useless, unsustainable, and often expensive "solutions."

Myth #1- Diet and Exercise Are the Key to Weight Loss

Let me begin this section by clearly stating that diet and exercise are indeed the stimuli for losing weight. The quality and amount of food you put into your body minus the amount of energy you spend moving your body is the equation that leads to weight loss. I am not arguing otherwise. What I am suggesting is that your past failures had little to do with diet and exercise knowledge. Knowing what to eat or what exercises to do or what piece of equipment you should (or shouldn't) be using has nothing to do with your barriers to success.

With that disclaimer out of the way, let's start with a few essential statistics. The obesity rate has grown fivefold in North America since the 1960's. The total weight loss spending market in North America is estimated to be five trillion dollars. In the span of fewer than 50 years, our weight loss product and service spending has grown almost tenfold. Even though our spending on education, products, services, and programs for losing weight has increased by 1000% in the last 50 years, our rate of obesity has continued to skyrocket. The more we learn, spend, and try to diet and exercise our way out of our weight problems, the more weight we gain.

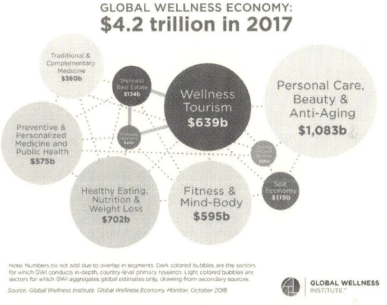

GLOBAL WELLNESS ECONOMY:
$4.2 trillion in 2017

Traditional & Complementary Medicine **$360b**

Wellness Real Estate **$134b**

Wellness Tourism **$639b**

Personal Care, Beauty & Anti-Aging **$1,083b**

Preventive & Personalized Medicine and Public Health **$575b**

Healthy Eating, Nutrition & Weight Loss **$702b**

Fitness & Mind-Body **$595b**

Spa Economy **$119b**

Note: Numbers do not add due to overlap in segments. Dark colored bubbles are the sectors for which GWI conducts in-depth, country-level primary research. Light colored bubbles are sectors for which GWI aggregates global estimates only, drawing from secondary sources.

Source: Global Wellness Institute, Global Wellness Economy Monitor, October 2018

GLOBAL WELLNESS INSTITUTE™

That might not be mind-blowing information, but what if you took those same metrics and applied them to some other area of expected improvement? What would you think about it then? Let's say your local police budget is 10 million dollars per year, and in the last 5 years, the crime rate has doubled. Your community government intervenes and says, "We are going to triple our spending to 30 million dollars per year to solve this problem! We are going to hire more officers, buy more guns, and double the amount of on-duty officers at any given time!" This, of course, is at the expense of the local taxpayers, which is money well spent if it solves a serious crime issue. Now imagine that over the next year the crime rate grows 300%. As a rational person, do you believe that the solution to crime is more police officers, more guns, and a further tax increase? I would hope not. You would consider the approach to be a complete failure. Well, that's the same way you should view the diet and exercise focus and spending that is growing year after year in the hopes of turning around the obesity epidemic. It. Is. Not. Working.

This is especially true when you consider the fact that diet and exercise information availability and education are now everywhere with unlimited access and excess. You can hop online and find 10,000 free diet and exercise methods to follow on any given day. If the key to weight loss were simply to know what to eat and what exercises to do, you wouldn't see a single overweight individual. This is, of course, not the reality of the situation.

The real reason we are collectively overweight and unhealthy runs much deeper than ideas as superficial as not knowing what to eat or what exercises to do, but more on that in the next chapter.

Myth #2- If we can't stick to diet and exercise efforts 100% of the time, we are weak and uncommitted

This is the most common belief of both fitness professionals and their struggling clients that is preventing any potential (and necessary) change in the weight loss industry. Chances are you've experienced these thoughts and feelings first hand. From a fitness professional's perspective, diet and exercise success is just a matter of eating well and exercising. They can do it, so their clients should be able to suck it up and do it too. The formula is simple. From the client's perspective, if we can't stick to the diet and exercise advice we are given, it is because we are uniquely weak and undisciplined. There are fit people in this world. If we aren't one of them, what other explanation can we have aside from fit people being healthy and disciplined and fat people being weak?

The problem with this thinking is it assumes the person who is trying to lose weight doesn't value their health. It also assumes that he or she doesn't have the willpower of a healthy, fit person. Let's start with the first assumption, as it is the easiest one to bust. There is not a single person on the face of this planet (whether he or she is willing to voice it or not) who wants to be overweight and unhealthy. There is not a single obese, sick person in this world who doesn't want to change their current health reality. To believe otherwise is quite frankly idiotic. Let's stop accepting the idea that when people fall off their diet and exercise plan, it is because they just don't care.

The second assumption that a lack of willpower is to blame is a more complex myth to destroy, but it is equally silly. When an overweight individual compares himself to someone who is "in shape", the common assumption is that the "in shape" person has rock-solid willpower, and the overweight person has none. This seems entirely logical, especially when you consider that diet and exercise changes are just a series of daily choices you either make or don't make. If you make the correct choices, you succeed. If you make the incorrect choices, you fail. But here is the thing about willpower: nobody has very much of it at all. Willpower is finite at best and non-existent at worst in all people, not just the ones who are struggling to lose weight. If you want to understand why and how this is true, you need to look into a concept called "ego depletion." The idea of ego depletion goes as follows: you begin your day with a limited amount of choice-making ability. That ability lessens with every decision you make and every stress you face. And these don't have to be important choices or pressures either. Deciding what clothes to wear in the morning, for example, requires depletion of your tiny vault of precious will. By the time the average person has rushed to work, fought with a co-worker, sworn at a fellow driver, and made the long commute back home, there is nothing left to prevent them from eating an entire box of cookies. This is an act that will temporarily help them forget about how lousy their day was. There is no more willpower left to reinforce wise decision-making.

You might be thinking, "If we all suffer from this ego depletion thing, how can there be any people in this world who are not overweight?" That's a good question, and we will begin to uncover the answer to it in the next chapter.

Myth #3- If I stick to diet and exercise efforts but don't lose weight, it is because I am genetically cursed to my overweight fate.

This myth is quickly rising in today's society. Still, it is also the easiest one to bust due to a precise scientific fact. If you remember the graph that charted the rise in obesity over the last 50-60 years, you'll remember that the rate of obesity has risen fivefold during that time. 50-60 years may seem like a significant period to a single human being. Still, when you compare it to the entire history of the modern human being, it is a blink of an eye. Why is this important? Here is the thing about genes: they need thousands (if not hundreds of thousands) of years to make a significant change to our biology. In fact (as you can see in the following image), our most notable biological changes take millions of years to evolve. That means that for our genetics to have evolved us into a community of genetically cursed overweight people, we would need at least a handful of millennia. So you must ask yourself the question, "If obesity was non-existent 100 years ago, but it takes thousands of years to alter your genetics, how can genetics be responsible for the acute rise in obesity?" I am sure you've gathered that it can't.

I am not suggesting weight loss isn't easier for some than others. It is. Some of us have a harder time finding exercise motivation. Some of us have lower base metabolisms and/or don't assimilate nutrition very well (assimilation is the converting of food into usable energy and nutrients). But (and this is a big but), it has been proven quite clearly that these genetic variations have a minor impact. So much so that in controlled studies, these variations did not prevent the study participants from losing adequate amounts of weight. For instance, when diet and exercise environments were in 100% control of the experimenters, all of the study participants were able to lose significant amounts of weight, regardless of the potential genetic differences. To summarize, genetics can play a small role in your fitness, but not to the degree of cursing you with obesity, and not to the point of being responsible for a rapid obesity crisis. Something else is going on here.

At this point in the book, you don't have to understand what you need to do to finally lose weight and be healthy. We still have more digging to go into why it is so hard for you to succeed (and there will be much more on that in the next few chapters). What is essential at this point is that you understand the 3 big myths that prevent us from grasping the real barriers between you and success. I hope I have done an adequate job of convincing you of these realities. For you to understand what the problem is as well as what your solution is going to be, you must acknowledge that diet and exercise is not the problem. When you can't make healthy choices, it is not because you are weak. And obesity rates in North America are not rising the way they are because we are genetically cursed. If you can agree with my argument against those common misconceptions, you are ready to understand what is really going on in your health.

Key Takeaways

· *The approach to weight loss is wrong because the problem is not adequately understood*
· *Diet and exercise lead to success only when the proper psychological foundation has been built*
· *We focus on '1% issues' and avoid the meaningful actions that make a big impact. This is because the 1% is simple and easy and the 99% is complex and difficult*

We bang our heads against the wall because we live in a diet and exercise culture that obsesses over what we eat and how we move without considering what drives our behaviour. While diet and exercise are indeed the stimuli for physical change, we cannot make those changes in any long-term way without addressing the driving forces behind unhealthy choices. We don't want to pull back the curtain on what is deep within our minds, so we keep looking for the next pill or diet trend, neither of which has ever worked in the past.

CHAPTER 2A: THE PRIMAL PARADOX

"An evolutionary perspective predicts that most diets and fitness programs will fail, as they do, because we still don't know how to counter once-adaptive primal instincts to eat donuts and take the elevator."
— Daniel E. Lieberman, The Story of the Human Body: Evolution, Health, and Disease

What would you say if I told you that obesity is the natural state of a human being? When you consider the history of our evolution, this is true. In fact, I don't believe the current rate of overweight and obese populations requires an explanation. What requires explanation is how any person manages to be fit and healthy in the modern world. The reason for my unique perspective on this matter begins with the primal paradox. The primal paradox is a term I use to describe what has happened to humans who evolved during times of scarcity but now live in times of great abundance. The vast majority of modern human beings fall under this category.

Depending on what you believe, human beings have been around a long time. The remains of human beings that are anatomically identical to modern humans have been dated back between 100,000 and 300,000 years. In other words, our bodies and brains have not fundamentally changed in the last 300,000 years. You might be asking yourself what that has to do with being overweight. The human body, as we know it today, was not developed in the last hundred or even thousand years. Our bodies and brains have evolved over millions of years, driven by what we needed to survive and reproduce at various points in human history. Today we are a product of the genetic adaptations that gave us the best chance of reproductive survival. Some of those evolved features still help us thrive, but we have also retained features that are now hurting our health. Everything from overeating at meals to general laziness can be traced back to our scarcity driven evolution. Daniel Lieberman labeled these adverse health outcomes as "evolutionary mismatches" in his book, The Story of the Human Body. Poor eyesight, cavities, certain kinds of cancers, and type 2 diabetes are all connected to evolutionary mismatches.

I hope the introduction I have given on this concept is clear, but to be safe, I will include a story. You must understand how evolutionary mismatches affect modern human beings in harmful ways. If you think you have a solid grasp on this concept, feel free to skip ahead.

The Story of Doug

Doug is a simple Sapiens. He lives in a nice-sized cave with a few stone carvings and walls covered with parietal art. When he is tired, he sleeps on a rug made from the skin of his latest kill. Like most of us, Doug spends each day doing the same things. He wakes when the sun rises, performs a few stretches in his cave bed, and begins his day.

Doug spends the first 3-4 hours of each day hunting and gathering the family provisions. When he isn't doing this, he is usually chewing, swallowing, and digesting whatever roots and tubers other members of his tribe located from the forest floor. If Doug is lucky, he will spend less time chewing hard roots and more time enjoying some berries or cooked meat. When he isn't hunting, gathering, or eating, Doug is usually lounging around and conserving as much energy as possible.

Sometimes life can be a little more exciting around camp. On a bad day, someone might get chased up a tree or into a hole by a fierce, hungry predator. In situations like this, an acute stress response allows Doug and his friends to react to danger and often survive. On a good day, Doug gets to take part in the act of reproduction, which we can assume was as much fun then as it is today. *I would omit the previous sentence entirely as it does not add information and cheapens your argument.* For the most part, the caveman life consists of a little bit of hunting, a little bit of gathering, and a little bit of eating.

Doug and his tribe spend so much time looking for food because it is both scarce and sometimes dangerous to attain. Cave people don't have the luxury of grocery stores or refrigeration, so every day they need to find new sources of sustenance. This way of life has brought upon a few evolutionary mechanisms that have made it easier for the tribe to survive. Doug and his friends have insatiable cravings for sugar, fat, and other high energy foods. If someone can find a pot of honey or a big fatty animal, the tribe has an ideal energy source for the week. But getting stung by bees or gored by a Buffalo is a severe deterrent. For this reason, craving systems have been designed to motivate the hunting and gathering of such foods.

The members of the tribe also like to take it easy when there isn't something to eat or a predator to run from. Why would they go through all the trouble of finding food, facing danger, or spending hours chewing roughage just to burn all the consumed energy? For this reason, laziness and energy conservation are critical during tribal downtime. If you took a human being from 100,000 years ago and put him or her into today's world, they would think we were crazy. Purposely avoiding high-calorie food that is in reach, or spending your free time going to a gym and intentionally burning calories would be a real head-scratcher. In fact, the original human being would envy the amount of body fat that most of us carry on our waists. Body fat equals survival and reproduction, and this is the driving force behind all animals, including humans.

I'm sure you've figured this out, but you are Doug. You have the same psychological and physiological driving forces as a cave person. What you *don't* have is the environment in which those tools are necessary for survival. This is the critical takeaway of this chapter. The evolutionary driving forces that kept us alive for hundreds of thousands of years were developed during times of scarcity. In those times, those tools served our ancestors very well, in fact well enough to make us the most dominant species in recordable history. The downside of this Darwinian evolution is that we now live in an environment that has become maladaptive. A scarcity built human is great for times of poverty, but in the modern world of abundance, this is now a big problem. This is the Primal Paradox.

We have intense cravings for sugar, fat, and other high-energy foods. If we can find a combination of all three (sugar, fat, and calories), that's the holy grail.

But now we have access to thousands of calories within 30 steps of any direction at all times. To make matters worse, our food has been agriculturally modified to be in the sweetest, fattiest, most energy-dense form possible. We are left with intense cravings for rare foods that are supposed to be hard to get our hands on. But now, they exist in our fridge, cupboard, and desk drawer. I'm sure you see the issue here.

It gets worse. Although what is known as the "thrifty gene" is debated in the world of science, there is no denying that human beings are very efficient at fat storage. When food was scarce, food waste was not an option. You ate every calorie that you had access to when the opportunity to eat presented itself. This is one of the main reasons why we now overeat at meals and typically consume everything that is on our plates, regardless of when we reach the point of fullness. The problem back then was that you could only use a finite amount of calories.

For this reason, our bodies intelligently evolved to take all extra calories we digest and stick them to our waist and thighs in the form of stored fat. We still store fat incredibly efficiently. Only now we have such an excess of caloric intake that we are storing fat to the point that it is killing us. Every calorie that is not used for an immediate biological function is stored as body fat. That's a great back-up system for when you might go a few days, a week, or even a month without food. But when access to calories is infinite, the fat stores continue to grow into excess.

This brings us to energy conservation. As mentioned earlier, there isn't much point in seeking out high-energy foods if you're just going to burn off all of the calories you consume. So when hunting, defending, or mating aren't happening, it is wise to shut things down and rest. This is what we know as "laziness." Modern human beings are still more likely to sit than stand. We are more motivated to watch TV than we are to exercise. Practices like taking the escalator instead of the stairs to conserve energy are driven by our default setting. Exercise is innately uncomfortable for people because recreational exercise would've moved you one step closer to death on the savannah. Exercise, as we know it today, was only used for essential activities during our most critical evolutionary periods. For this reason, most people have a slight distaste for random acts of exercise. When movement is not serving a crucial purpose, we are happy to lay around and watch Netflix.

If all that isn't enough, here is the kicker. The stress response that kept our ancestors from being eaten by predators remains with us in a problematic way. This is the same response that spikes our blood sugar and fires up our cortisol when we face daily stress. The problem is that we no longer utilize these hormonal responses to escape from predators. Well, most of us don't, I assume. These days we are being chased by debt, disease, and chronic sources of anxiety instead. This results in unfavourable hormonal cascades that circulate in our bloodstream far too often, and the result is killing us.

To summarize, problems like cravings, overeating, fat storage, laziness, and stress used to serve us well. In fact, these were essential functions for human survival. That is why they are so strongly represented in the modern human brain. Unfortunately, we now live in a world where these driving forces have become problematic, and we aren't evolving away from them any time soon.

What I want you to understand above all else is that your problems are not unique. They are not specific to you. The primal drivers that push you into your worst behaviours have nothing to do with your personality. This is important to understand because we often feel isolated in our weight problems. We feel as though we are choosing to be unhealthy due to internal weakness or commitment issues. This is unhelpful. Making long-lasting changes in your daily habits and behaviours is hard work. If every time you eat a few slices of pizza or a little too much ice cream, you become self-hating, you're never going to stick around long enough to succeed. It just hurts too badly.

I want to be clear that I am not giving you permission to let your health slide. While the primal paradox is a genuine issue, it does not remove your personal responsibility from the matter. It might not be your fault that you struggle to lose weight and be healthy, but it's still up to you to do something about it. If a reasonable amount of human beings have found a way to overcome the primal paradox and its evolutionary mismatches, you can do the same.

Before moving onto the next chapter, I want you to know that there is indeed a way to take control of the primal paradox and your health. I say this because a part of you may feel a bit discouraged after hearing that you are designed to be heavy. If we are intended to be fat and lazy, what's the point in trying? There is a solution, but we need to understand each problem before we get into the solution. I believe this is critical. For the time being, do your best to absorb the information I am introducing and begin taking note of how these issues show up in your own life. Doing so will leave you prepared to properly implement your personal solution when we get to that section of the book. For now, let's move on to our toxic culture.

Key Takeaways

- *Obesity isn't abnormal. Good health is.*
- *An old brain combined with the modern world is the driving force behind most modern unhealthy actions*
- *It would be best if you were forgiving of your bad habits, but not complacent when it comes to changing them*
- *Your worst behaviours are not a matter of character, so self-hatred is unhelpful at best, and at worst, a barrier between you and success*

The primal paradox is a double-edged sword. On the one hand, it can feel defeating to understand that you are biologically designed to fail. On the other hand, this reality should leave you more forgiving of your missteps. The number one reason why people fail is that we take unhealthy behaviour personally. Overeating, snacking, and laziness are not a matter of character, so stop letting habits defeat you. If you can take this view and change your inward attitude, everything becomes more manageable.

Chapter 2B- Our Toxic Culture

Mainstream medical practice largely ignores the role of emotions in the physiological functioning of the human organism. Yet the scientific evidence abundantly shows that people's lifetime emotional experiences profoundly influence health and illness. And, since emotional patterns are a response to the psychological and social environment, disease in an individual always tells us about the multigenerational family of origin and the broader culture in which that person's life unfolds .

- Dr.Gabor Mate

In the previous co-chapter, we looked at the subconscious motivations that drive us to seek out high-energy foods, overeat, and be lazy. This is the maladaptive process that I refer to as the Primal Paradox: the problematic result of humans designed for scarcity now living in abundance. The key takeaway from the chapter is that as a human being, your food and exercise-related behavioural issues are by design. If you can see this principle playing out in your own life, there isn't anything else you need to know about your evolutionary mismatches.

In this chapter, we will look into how our toxic modern environment (and culture) maximizes the problems born out of the Primal Paradox. We will look at how modern manufactured foods, government guidelines, educational institutions, and social media seem to exacerbate an already harmful internal conflict. As in previous chapters, I will use a few stories to help you connect with the core issue of this section. If you would prefer to skip it and get to the "meat" of the matter, you are welcome to do so.

The Story of Jessica (and the media that harms her)

Jessica is your average thirty-something female. She has a good group of friends, a supportive and loving family, and a job that brings stability and satisfaction to her life. What Jessica is lacking, however, is in the department of her physical and mental wellbeing.

Over the years, Jessica has not just grown in age. She has also grown in pant sizes. She hasn't gained a dramatic amount of weight, but she is steadily moving in the wrong direction on the scale, and it bothers her. Jessica has never been what she would consider "skinny", and for most of her life, she didn't worry about her weight. In fact, she never negatively thought about her body until her mid-twenties. If you asked those close to Jessica, they wouldn't have even noticed or acknowledged her weight gain. So why does this modest change seem to be now walloping Jessica?

As Jessica matured, joined the workforce, and became increasingly routine, she also started to value her downtime. She doesn't go out very much during the week and is very much a homebody. She reserves social events for the weekend and doesn't dare leave the house at night from Monday to Friday. Most days, Jessica comes home after work, makes dinner, cleans up around the house, and then "unwinds." Unwinding might include some PVR'd daytime T.V., a few gossip magazines, or some time spent on her laptop to check Instagram or Facebook.

There's a common theme between the media that Jessica consumes each evening. She will inevitably come across a female figure who makes her feel inferior in one way or another. When Jessica watches her T.V. show, it often features the latest celebrity weight loss trend. When she reads her gossip magazines, they are filled with glamorous shots of the world's most "beautiful" people. Either that or harsh criticisms of these same people if the paparazzi can catch them in an unflattering beach picture. "Wasn't Kim Kardashian featured as one of People Magazine's most beautiful people 6 months ago, and now this month she 'hasn't recovered well' from her latest pregnancy"?

Lastly, when Jessica checks out social networks, it's even worse. Everyone from friends to internet fitness models to celebrities she follows seem to be slim and fabulous. Filters, professional airbrushing, and other tricks of the trade make it impossible to know if she is looking at real human beings. Only the best photos taken with the best lighting of life's most perfect moments are on display.

After a 3-hour long media blitz, Jessica can't help but feel a little overweight. It seems as though everyone has it together and she is physically falling apart. Jessica is not what you would consider a particularly sensitive person. She is, by all means, as mentally secure as anyone else. In fact, before Jessica fell into the world of social media, she didn't even notice any sort of "weight issue." But for some reason, she can't help but be negatively affected by what she sees in all the various forms of media she consumes each day. Worse, she can't escape it even though she knows that it is hurting her psychologically. She is a glutton for the pain, seemingly addicted to the self-image of others. She is resentful of her friends when she sees the picture-perfect lives and bodies they portray on social networks, but she can't stop looking at their accounts. A girl who was once a resilient and confident woman is now lacking self-worth and mental stability. Jessica's toxic culture has pushed her into insecurity and emotional turmoil. Is Jessica overweight and in need of some sort of dietary intervention, or has the toxicity of popular media made her see herself differently when she looks in the mirror? I'll let you decide.

The Story of Rick (and how we treat dysfunctional lifestyles)

Rick is your average North American male. He works hard, takes care of his family, and has his own methods of "decompression." He likes beer and burgers with his sports, and he watches a lot of games. When it comes to working, Rick has a fairly stressful job. He works long hours and has endless responsibility. He manages over 100 employees and oversees his company's union. With the constant threat of layoffs and sending jobs overseas or having positions filled by robots, the thought of unemployment is always looming in Rick's mind. The stress of work has brought on a constant need to escape and unwind with food and media. The direct consequence is a steadily growing beer belly and noticeable changes in energy and feelings of wellbeing. Indirectly, the stress of work and the constant need to escape is affecting Rick's life in other dangerous ways. He has been fighting with his wife frequently. They both seem to be irritable and perpetually resentful of one another. It has gotten to the point that the only time they communicate is by attacking one another or being passive-aggressive. Life is not getting any easier, and Rick is suffering in many ways.

Before the age of forty, Rick could drink a 12 pack, eat a few cheeseburgers, and watch 4-6 hours of football without it noticeably affecting his health. He's had a steadily growing "beer belly" for the better part of the last decade, and he can no longer deny its existence. What's of more significant concern is that Rick is beginning to notice some symptoms that he hasn't experienced before. He seems to get easily fatigued, sometimes barely being able to get out of bed. He finds himself getting dizzy for no apparent reason and needing to sit down more often. The most annoying thing of all is that he is getting up to urinate several times each night. Rick knows that something is just not *right*.

Eventually, the concerns become so overwhelming that Rick finally goes to see his family doctor, something most men rarely do. The doctor listens to Rick's growing list of symptoms and concerns and decides to run diagnostics. Not surprisingly, Rick's results come back with high blood pressure, cholesterol concerns, and borderline diabetic blood glucose readings. This isn't anything that Rick's doctor hasn't seen before, and many of these results he considers to be 'normal' for an aging man.

Rick's doctor puts him on a handful of prescription drugs to help alleviate and control his symptoms, and Rick is sent home. There isn't any discussion about diet, activity level, stress levels, or any other lifestyle factors. In fairness to the physician, he only has 10 minutes to spend with Rick, and in the doctor's experience, diet and exercise advice fall on deaf ears. So Rick leaves the office with a prescription for four different medications and permission to continue down a road of overwhelming stress and self-destruction.

The Story of Annie (and how we derive value only from what we produce)

Annie is a professional woman. She works at a prestigious law firm and is feared by many in her field. She thrives on being seen as a "shark." Annie is a defence lawyer who spends her days defending dangerous criminals: murderers, rapists, and pedophiles. She has the kinds of social interactions that leave her a colder human being.

Annie has always considered herself to be a strong

woman, so much so that she is continually aiming to prove her strengths. She can be abrasive and always appears to be ready for a fight. Perhaps it is more accurate to say that she lives for legal battles. Despite all that, Annie's once sharp mind and body are becoming frail. It seems that in a matter of a few months, she has started to become a shell of her once fierce identity.

Annie has been crying at night, uncontrollably for the last month. She doesn't know why. Nothing in her life has changed, and she can't pin her grief on any specific event. When she gets home, she just sits down and cries. It is as if overwhelming emotion crashes over her like a giant wave, and she begins to drown in it.

While Annie has not had any dangerous thoughts or taken part in any self-harming behaviour during this time, she *is* seeing herself in a negative light. She feels weak. Annie feels like she is becoming everything the kids at school used to call her.

Concerned about her condition, Annie goes to see a psychiatrist who was highly recommended by a friend. After her first week of sessions, Dr. Moss writes Annie a prescription for antidepressants and sleeping pills. His immediate concern is getting Annie's psychological symptoms under control so she can function day to day. The complex roots of her condition will take time to uncover, but for now, pills might help. Annie will continue with weekly follow-ups, and for the time being the prescriptions will hopefully relieve her psychological pain.

A few weeks into the medication Annie feels arguably better. She hasn't had any of the devastating lows that she was experiencing prior, and that is very comforting. She is operating more effectively at the law firm, and she is regaining her confidence. But at what cost? Annie doesn't feel much of anything at all. She doesn't feel love or affection, and her empathy has disappeared. This works well for a defence lawyer, but is it a positive state of mind for a mother, sister, wife, or friend?

The Jamison Family (and the common struggle toward healthy eating)

It is Tuesday after school, and Cheryl Jamison is on her way to pick her kids up from school. All five of them. Her husband, Mike, works 12-14 hour days at the plant, so after her afternoon shift at the local drug mart, Cheryl rushes to get the kids.

Tuesday is grocery day, so before going home, the Jamisons stop at the local grocery store to get food for the week. This experience usually requires significant amounts of math and well thought out purchases because the family is on a tight budget. Cheryl begins by taking the children through the whole foods section with the best of intentions. Bell peppers are six dollars a pound, raspberries are seven dollars a pint, and the cheapest cut of red meat is $8.99 per lb. On the other hand, there is the boxed and canned foods section. Sugary breakfast cereal, chips, pop, and other heavily subsidized processed foods are two dollars a box and five for five dollars. Cheryl knows that the whole foods are healthier, but she also knows that she can stretch her budget much farther in the pre-packaged section. Not only that, but the sugar-laden processed foods are the ones that the kids are begging for. Even three-year-old Carl, her youngest, can recognize the cartoon character from his favorite T.V. show on the cereal box.

By the time the Jamisons get to check out, they have a full cart of foods that fit into their family budget, but not a vegetable or even fresh fruit in sight. Maybe next week there will be some more sales, but for right now, this will have to do.

What is the point of these three stories? This is not intended to be an attack on the medical system or to be used to remove the personal responsibility that comes with social media or food selection. It is clear to me, however, that we have systematic cultural issues that drive people into disease states.

In Jessica's story, I am highlighting the negative images and messaging that are now supercharged in social media. Popular media is leading to feelings of low self-worth in both men and women. Constant social comparison to ridiculous standards of beauty and "manliness" is driving both sexes, young and old, into pits of deep insecurity.

In Rick's story, I am highlighting the emotional drain on modern workers as well as a broken medical system that prescribes in place of investigating. This is by design and not the fault of first-line physicians. It is the result of the relationship between educational institutions, drug companies, and government health care.

In Annie's story, I am highlighting how we derive human value from what we produce, not who we are. We are the "rise and grind" generation that envies those who work 16 hours a day to drive the $100,000 car. I also touch on the decline of mental health and the potential consequences of medicating issues that are emotionally driven.

Lastly, in the Jamisons' story, I touched on how our subsidization of processed foods is forcing the average family to make unhealthy decisions. I also included a quick note regarding the irresponsible marketing of food companies toward children.

When it comes to our weight, we usually focus on surface-level biology. We believe that what we eat and how we exercise determines our waistline. The reality is that health problems are culturally and socially driven. Have you considered how your social stresses, financial anxieties, and adverse life experiences have motivated you to self-medicate your mind with unhealthy actions? Have you thought about how societal factors like beauty standards and social media lead you to attach your worth to your weight and make you hate yourself? These psychological and societal factors are driving you to eat, and be too self-conscious to take care of yourself at the most basic level.

If you want to begin changing your life, you need to get past the focus on genetics, body type, metabolism, and all the like. If you are overweight, there are social and psychological contributors that are making your problem harder to deal with. It is all connected.

Biology is definitely a factor in our health and fitness. Hormonal issues, the ability to gain muscle mass, and our internal motivation for exercise have all been linked to genetic factors. But these issues rarely lead to weight gain by themselves, at least not weight gain that cannot be controlled or reversed. Psychological problems like being sensitive to stress, being sad or frustrated, having a poor self-image, and rationalizing your unhealthy actions are the x-factors. If you grow up in a society where fast food, sugary drinks, excessive drinking, and binge T.V. watching are considered normal, you're going to struggle. If you are exposed to unrealistic beauty standards at a young age, you will have a distorted idea of what "healthy" looks like. The cards are stacked against you.

What I am hoping you will take away from this chapter is that you have been raised, and live in, a toxic culture. Mental and physical health is an uphill battle that is not supported by the government, medicine, educational institutions, or popular media. Unfortunately, these are the organizations to which we are regularly exposed, and that influence us. Your sense of value, your sense of beauty, and your sense of what it means to thrive have been under attack since you were old enough to look at a T.V. screen.

When you combine this with the primal paradox, it is no wonder that you have struggled so long to eat right and make exercise stick.

CHAPTER 3: ADVERSE LIFE EXPERIENCES, STRESS, AND SELF-MEDICATION

"To further complicate the issue of obesity: while genes do exist that predispose people to weight gain, we now also have a food system that produces food that "soothes" us in all the wrong ways (AKA "junk food", "processed food", etc.) by feeding into our neuro-hormonal system of desire and reward. The more traumatized we are, the more we desire toxic, addictive foods, the more we gain weight and the more vulnerable our brains become... and the vicious cycle continues."

Why do we eat when we are stressed? Why do we watch hours of television with a bowl of chips in our lap when sad? When we are suffering from anxiety or anger, why do we turn to alcohol or some other numbing, distractive agent?

The first two barriers discussed have uncovered problematic mechanisms in both our lower, primal brains and our higher, modern minds. The combination of these has left us with an immediate health disadvantage. The explanation of the primal paradox and our toxic culture tells us a lot about the aspects of human history that hurt our health. The topic of this third barrier, however, concerns your own personal life history. We are moving away from the generalized human disadvantages we face and toward your unique set of problems. To continue with the theme of this book, I'd like to introduce the concept of this chapter with a short story.

The Story of Jenny

Jenny is an average 35-year-old woman. She has a family who loves her, friends who care for her, and many of life's other securities. Like many women her age, however, Jenny is becoming less satisfied with her weight and appearance. She does not have a significant other, and according to her well-meaning (but often cruel) mother, if she just lost a few pounds and took better care of herself, she'd have a boyfriend by now.

Jenny is active. She walks a few times each week, plays at a charity lawn bowling tournament on Thursday nights, and tries to get to the gym at least once per week. But thus far, none of her efforts, modest as they may be, seem to make any difference in her body.

Although Jenny tries to be as healthy as possible, there are unhealthy habits that she just can't kick. The big ones for her are late-night snacking and red wine consumption. Despite Jenny's best efforts, she cannot put down the cookie bag or the wine bottle between the hours of 8pm and midnight.

There's a clear pattern to her evenings. After dinner, she putters around the house doing some light cleaning and organizing, and then without much else to do, she ends up sitting on the couch and turning on the T.V. This is when the cookies and wine start calling her name. Jenny initially resists these sugar and alcohol-based urges, reminding herself that she is trying to cut back on indulgences, but after about 5 minutes of mental anguish, she gives in. She tells herself that it'll be "just a few cookies and a small glass of red wine. I deserve it today!" An hour later, Jenny has consumed 4 glasses of wine and ½ of the bag of cookies. She feels sick to her stomach, guilty, ashamed, and all of the other usual feelings one would get after a night of losing control. As with most people, Jenny believes that this is the result of character flaws. Jenny sees herself as weak. She believes that she doesn't have any willpower. This is why she is fat, and this is why she is alone. Jenny routinely falls into this self-destructive headspace.

What Jenny doesn't consider is what is currently happening at work. Her new professional life has been causing her almost daily stress. It turns out that Jenny does have an interested suitor: her 64-year-old, married boss. For the better part of a year, despite her best efforts to show her lack of interest, Jenny's boss has proceeded to touch her and speak to her in inappropriate ways at work. The actions are not dangerous or aggressive, but clearly unacceptable. Jenny has repeatedly asked her boss to stop his advances, but in his assumption of power that he states could be used to ruin her career, he ignores her evident discomfort.

You may be asking yourself why Jenny does not just go and tell someone what is happening to her? Why doesn't she get him fired? Why doesn't she sue him for every penny he is worth? The truth is that Jenny feels powerless, and her boss (being the predator he is) knows it. All predators understand what to look for in a victim, and Jenny's boss is a master at this game.

Before pondering why Jenny doesn't put a stop to this situation, you must consider her past. Jenny was once in a similar situation with an "uncle", not a blood relative but a family friend who was close enough to be trusted alone with Jenny on occasion. When she was 12 years old, she experienced the same inappropriate touching, talking, and feelings of powerlessness from this man. She is now reliving this pain and helplessness in the workplace. The family friend's conduct was never dangerous in the sense of causing physical or sexual harm, but despite her young age, Jenny knew that the advances were not okay. During this earlier experience, why did Jenny not tell her parents what was happening? At the time, Jenny was afraid to shame her parents or threaten the relationship between her "uncle" and her father. This was the best man at her parent's wedding. How could she speak up if it meant ruining the family ties? Also, he was never shy about emphasizing all of the awful things that would happen if she told anyone about his conduct. Adult Jenny is still that same little girl who believes she needs to save everyone around her the pain of her trauma by just being quiet. So she will continue going to work and dealing with the inappropriateness of her boss in silence and hope that it one day stops.

You may be asking yourself what a situation like this has to do with being overweight. How does this sort of experience relate to unhealthy habits and behaviours? Very simply, your actions dictate your outcomes. This makes sense to most people. What fewer people understand is that your emotions (anger, sadness, fear, disgust) drive your actions. What only a minority of people realize is that adverse life experiences dictate your emotional sensitivities. Divorce, abuse, lack of acceptance, unsupportive parents, purposelessness, not having friends, bullying, and the like leave deep scars that we carry with us into adulthood. We suppress these pains, but they bubble up in the adult expression of anger, sadness, fear, and disgust. When, as adults, we are triggered into the emotions to which we are uniquely sensitive, we do whatever it takes to shut them down. Luckily for us, food, laziness, alcohol, and technological distraction are the most convenient, easily accessible, socially acceptable forms of self-medication on the market.

We all have unresolved issues from their past that stick with us as we continue on through life. This is why we get angry for inappropriate reasons. It's why looking in the mirror can make us sad. It's why most people have an underlying theme of anxiety in their daily life. We assume that the kind of adverse life event that could affect us negatively long into the future can only stem from the most sinister forms of abuse: physical and sexual. But less acutely painful or damaging life experiences can create deep defence systems that protect us in the short term but hurt us in the long run. "Trauma", as it is known, comes in many forms and along a broad spectrum of seriousness. Adverse events in life often determine how susceptible we are to unhealthy types of self-medication when faced with feelings and emotions we did not develop the tools to deal with healthily. As mentioned, life pain does not have to be as severe as the kind that Jenny is currently experiencing with her boss's sexual advances. Relationship issues, work stress, financial stress, health concerns, and even plain boredom can create more than enough internal discomfort to push us toward self-medication and coping. And what are the most readily available "drugs" we have access to for the purpose of self-medication? The answer is food, alcohol, sloth, and technology. While these possible sources of self-medication are vastly different from one another, they all have one thing in common: the ability to distract us from our emotions and temporarily numb us from the pain we feel.

Let's take this concept and go back to Jenny's story to connect the example to real life. Jenny is sensitive to male relationships due to her early life experiences. These were worsened by feeling helpless and needing to stay quiet. Remember that Jenny kept the events to herself out of fear that bringing forward the abuse would upset her parents. Jenny became the protector of her parents. Now, as an adult, Jenny is facing a similar situation with her boss. Since she is already highly sensitive to abusive male relationships, the adverse effects of her boss's unwelcome advances leave her feeling more helpless than another grown woman would who has not experienced this behaviour before. Most women in her situation would have spoken out and sought out support. The combination of her underlying sensitivity (past abuse) and the current pain she is facing (workplace sexual harassment) has created a series of significant emotional pains that she hadn't developed tools to deal with in a healthy way. So Jenny self-medicates with food and alcohol at the end of the day when her idle mind opens her up to overwhelming pain and discomfort. Much like a drug addict who continues to abuse substances even though they know this is slowly killing them, Jenny continues to self-medicate although she knows it's not healthy because she seeks immediate pain relief. Sensitivity (adverse life experiences) multiplied by pain (emotional distress) drives coping (food and alcohol). Jenny is merely trying to make herself feel better. More accurately, she is trying to distract herself from her current pain.

The case of Jenny is somewhat extreme, though not uncommon. I am guessing most readers of this book were not sexually abused at a young age and are not currently experiencing blatant sexual harassment at work. But her story clearly illustrates my point. Jenny's example might leave you sitting there and thinking to yourself, "I was never abused, nor am I currently being abused, and I still get lost in a bag of cookies and bottle of wine most nights." The causes of sensitivity and pain do not have to be extreme to lead us into food and drink self-medication that results in weight problems. Extreme examples highlight the process. In many cases, the most sinister forms of abuse leave such a painful mark in the victim's mind that those who face them end up with severe drug and alcohol abuse issues. While drugs and alcohol can be the necessary escape for those who have suffered the worst atrocities, food is the drug of choice for people who may not even realize they are emotionally bruised.

Let's say you were bullied as a child. Not violently, but perhaps you moved to a new school and didn't fit in. You didn't have a place in your new school where you felt socially secure or where you felt like you could be yourself and still have good friendships. An entire school year of name-calling, fear, and a growing distaste for going to school can fester into an inability to properly cope with social stress. Because you are facing a novel amount of social anxiety for a young boy or girl, you build unnatural self-defence mechanisms to get by. Even if you grow up to become confident and have lots of friends, you are still likely to be sensitive to specific social stressors in adult life. So now, as an adult, when you have interpersonal issues at work or at home, you suffer more than a person who did not develop that same childhood sensitivity. When you face those social stressors in adulthood, you do not cope with them well, and you are driven to self-medicate.

An example of this is the person who has to have food or drink in hand at a party. Someone who has struggled with social issues at a young age will be far more likely to gravitate toward the consumption of alcohol and the occupation of their hands and mouth with food to feel less exposed. You depend on the alcohol to quiet the social anxiety in your head and the food to occupy your hands and mouth. This helps an anxious person who is always feeling judged avoid the feelings of social awkwardness. A child who grew up in a socially secure environment with close friends and no bullying isn't likely to require these crutches in adult situations.

Another example would be the over-stimulated child. Imagine if you grew up and never had imaginative downtime without access to your technology or toys. You grew up with gaming systems, T.V., movies, the internet, and you never knew what it was like to deal with boredom. Now in adulthood, when you are sitting around between dinner and bedtime wondering what you're going to do with yourself, you get painfully bored. Yes, boredom is a pain inside the brain. What's the easiest way to get rid of brain pain that stems from boredom? Habitual chewing, drinking, and technological distraction like T.V., Youtube, Netflix, and social networks. This is a common reason why many of us snack all night long, even though we are not hungry. The pain of boredom is so extreme that quieting our idle anxiety is more important than making healthy choices. Apathy also leaves us stuck with our thoughts. When we are not distracted, we are more susceptible to the daily emotional stresses that push us into unhealthy self-medication.

I hope you can see yourself in at least one of those three examples. Making these connections is the beginning of moderating your unhealthy behaviour.

Any past experience combined with any pain can lead to coping through food, drink, lethargy, or technological distraction. The combinations of triggers and coping mechanisms are endless. Below I have worked through a few examples to help you understand the connection.

1. You had a verbally abusive dad when you were a child. Now when you face male authority (like dealing with your boss at work), it pushes you

into high levels of stress and anger. You distract yourself from this pain with overeating and late-night snacking.

2. You had parents who used food to keep you quiet when you were growing up, almost like a surrogate babysitter. When you wanted stimulation and interaction, you got food shoved in your face. Now when you are unstimulated and bored, you are drawn to food to relieve the pain of the boredom.

3. When you were young, you never felt like you had anything in your life that you were great at. You felt like you didn't have a place in the world or anything of value to give. You felt like you didn't have a purpose. Now, as an adult, you don't feel as though your job is good enough. You are always comparing your life and career to those around you. You are left feeling as though everyone is ahead of you. These thoughts and feelings of worthlessness and lack of purpose push into alcohol consumption at night to distract you from these uncomfortable emotions.

Examples are not limited to this model. What I want you to grasp is the following. Any negative experience that you were not, at the time, emotionally equipped to deal with, has potentially resulted in a sensitivity and set of defence mechanisms that hurt you in adult life. When those past sensitivities are exposed to present pain, you will have trouble coping in a healthy way. Therefore, you end up seeking external coping methods. Food, drink, laziness, and technological distraction are the most readily available and socially acceptable forms of self-medication we have access to, and we use these to stimulate, numb, and distract. Most of the time, we aren't even conscious of the connection between our underlying pain and our unhealthy actions. We just assume that stress, anxiety, sadness, anger, frustration, helplessness, and worthlessness come with being an adult. We are disconnected from the roots of our unhealthy behaviours.

If you recall the first section of this book, you will remember my suggestion that the 60-year rise in obesity is not the result of a lack of diet and exercise resources. It is not the result of individual weakness or lack of willpower, or any significant genetic changes. So the question worth asking is what is the actual problem we are facing. I believe this is best answered by a brilliant author and personal mentor, Dr. Gabor Mate. Doctor Mate once said, "we do not have an obesity epidemic; we have a stress epidemic." Dr. Mate suggests that the cause of our uncontrolled searches for stimuli that lead us into overeating, intense cravings, lack of exercise, and several other barriers to quality health come from our need to self-medicate.

I know that this concept will be foreign to many readers. You might be thinking to yourself, "you're telling me that my diet or lack of exercise is not the problem, but rather it's the inner discomfort that pushes me to 'self- medicate' with unhealthy actions?" That is precisely what I am suggesting. By the end of the book, this will be proven. In fact, this point of view should not be controversial. To illustrate this, I am going to introduce you to the Food Relationship Origin and Sensitivity Test (FROST). I and a few Western university students designed the FROST test to show a connection between adverse life experiences and obesity. The hypothesis is that adverse life experiences, and lack of support when facing them, are directly related to a person's adult weight and health. Over 400 participants who were actively trying to take control of their health completed the survey. The results were compelling. For each instance of an adverse life event ranging from abuse to bullying to lack of purpose, or a lack of support in the form of resources, family values, or supportive parents, the participant's BMI increased by .33 points. That means a person who took the FROST test who experienced every adverse life event would have a BMI that was 13.2 points higher than someone who didn't experience any adverse life events. That is the difference between being a healthy weight and having class 2 obesity. This is incredibly significant.

The adverse events we face where we lack the tools to properly process them directly correlate to a heavier body. Adverse life experiences (or trauma) increase our sensitivity to present pain (often called stress), which drives us into unhealthy coping habits like overeating, snacking, alcohol consumption, and technological distraction. To demonstrate this process, I would like to insert a story about Kelly.

The Story of Kelly

Kelly has never managed stress well. As a child, she had to face many "catty" girls at school who made her life miserable daily. When she would tell her mother that she was having a tough time with her social life, her mother would simply tell her, "everyone gets bullied, and you'll get over it. Toughen up, Kelly." This unhelpful but typical response led Kelly to bottle up all of her fear and pain. Due to her mother's stoic responses, she didn't believe her suffering was worth mentioning to her parents anymore. Would you want to take your most concerning issues to someone who minimized them and left you feeling unsupported and misunderstood? Kelly's difficult school days, combined with a lack of understanding, supportive parents, prevented her from developing internal coping mechanisms for social stress. She had to learn to create her own defence mechanisms in place of healthier social tools. Time passed, and Kelly grew. As she got older, the school situation improved, and the bullying eventually subsided. Unfortunately, the damage to Kelly's internal stress management system was already done. When she got to college, she had a great time. Post secondary school was a blast, and Kelly excelled in a higher educational environment. She had lots of friends, and her confidence grew as she aged. After college, she got a job she wanted right away and loved her first year in the workforce. Kelly went through the majority of her early adult life 'stress-free' and seemingly unaffected by her old childhood anxieties. Then things began to change.

As is the case for most of us, as Kelly got older, life became increasingly serious. Demands at work started to grow beyond what she felt capable of managing. The once confident young professional began to question her abilities, and it showed in the workplace. As the work environment became more and more competitive, Kelly began to feel as though her co-workers were out to compete with her, not work collaboratively with her. She began to experience increasing conflicts with her superiors, who didn't seem to support her concern for the interpersonal work conflicts. At the end of the workday, Kelly came home stressed and exhausted. It was catching up with her. Sometimes she felt like these stresses could be remedied with a glass of red wine. Not an excessive amount, just enough to help her relax and decompress on the couch. On awful days she would add a croissant or some other piece of pastry into the mix. If it were a day from hell, she would add in one or two chocolate bars.

While these food and drink relaxation aids never made the problems disappear, they allowed Kelly to numb out for a little while. This feeling of numbness during hard times is what is commonly known as "taking the edge off."

As time passed, work didn't improve, nor did Kelly's decompression habits. The same amount of stress didn't seem to be remedied by the same amount of food or wine. Weeks went by, and Kelly was increasing her wine, pastry, and chocolate intake to the point that she was going to bed with a buzz and waking up with a stomach ache.

Kelly's Search for Dopamine

As you now know, the negative emotions that Kelly experiences are recognized in her mind as discomfort or pain. Stress, anger, frustration, helplessness, sadness, and boredom all say to the brain "Something is happening here that we don't like, let's do something about it." When the mind is experiencing discomfort, it looks to the dopamine reward system for fast relief. Many actions can cause an increase in the release of dopamine, but the most convenient and accessible dopamine trigger is highly palatable food. The dopamine reward system in our brain was designed to inspire us to take or avoid actions that kept us alive long enough to reproduce. This is an evolutionary mechanism that we discussed earlier in the book. Anytime we were able to find calorie-dense foods, our brain would fire up the dopamine reward system and make us feel good, either by stimulating, distracting, or numbing our minds. This response to behavioural reinforcement pushed us to seek out the foods that would allow us to stay alive, lay around in the shade, and have sex, when we weren't taking part in any necessary survival activities. This process of dopamine-based behavioural reinforcement kept us around long enough to spread our genes and expand the human race.

Dopamine reward mechanisms still live inside of our modern brain, but they have not evolved to deal with the amount of stimulation we readily provide them. During the necessary evolution of our dopamine reward system, we didn't have access to sugar, fat, comfort, technological distraction, or even mates like we do today. Since the dopamine response developed in times of scarcity, it is not equipped to be stimulated as often as is now necessary.

So what is the result of this mismatch, and what does it have to do with Kelly? Kelly is facing an incredible amount of stress she is not equipped to handle. This is due to the scarring left by early life bullying experiences and the lack of support from her parents. As a result, she seeks external sources of self-medication to manage her adult anxieties. At first, a small snack and a glass of red wine were enough to get her through the pain of her destructive emotional rumination. But when her brain became overstimulated with chocolate, croissants, and wine, she began to dull her dopamine receptors. For Kelly to get the same reward in the future, she required more "medication." The brain dulls the effects of the dopamine reward system, and the same amount of self-medication does not give the same amount of relief. If Kelly wants to numb or stimulate her way out of emotional distress, she will need to increase her food and alcohol intake. Food and wine have "hijacked" Kelly's dopamine reward system.

This process repeats itself over and over again. The more Kelly feeds her dopamine reward system with self-medicating behaviours, the duller her response becomes, and the more self-medicating she must do in the future to find comfort. This is a similar process to what leads to the eventual overdose in hard drug addicts. Addicts are fundamentally facing an extreme version of the same problem Kelly has. I don't say that to minimize the seriousness of drug addiction. If anything, it should help you to see yourself in those who are facing the most extreme pain in life. The same "fix" of the drug does not dull the pain for the addict the way it once did. S/he must then increase the dosage to get the same sense of relief. Over time, the dosage necessary for a response gets so high that the body cannot tolerate the toxicity of the drug. If you want to learn more about addiction, read Dr. Gabor Mate's book In the Realm of Hungry Ghosts.

You can see how this process of self-medicating your pain is happening inside of you every day. This is happening inside all of us. Still, different people self medicate with different things based on the intensity of their past life experiences, the resources they had to deal with those experiences, their current environment, and the pain that they experience each day. Whether a person gambles himself into massive debt, shops his way into bankruptcy, or drinks himself to death, the cycle is the same. Some people become drug addicts. Some people become workaholics. But the most common addiction and form of self-medication we see in the world today is the addiction to food, alcohol, technology, and sloth based distractions.

Why Now?

Human beings have arguably existed for hundreds of thousands (if not millions) of years. Why do we have an obesity crisis right now? I'm sure our grandparents and their parents had to deal with some pretty awful life experiences, so why is the obesity crisis happening in such recent history? The answer to that question is twofold. One hundred years ago, we didn't have the available medication we have now. We had very few stores to buy food. Now we have millions of calories available to us within a city block at all times. The modification of hyper-palatable, calorie-dense food is also a very modern food system. Food processing has allowed for increased taste and more significant sugar and fat concentrations in packaged foods. This has resulted in increased stimulation for the dopamine reward system per unit of food. Even fruits and vegetables are sweeter, larger, and more easily digested than their original forms. Our preferred food-based medication is stronger, cheaper, more available, and more harmful than it was even 30 years ago. Food manufacturers currently have teams of scientists whose sole purpose is to figure out how to formulate foods that keep consumers coming back.

The second cause of the recent crisis in obesity is our toxic culture. We face such incredible amounts of stress with so few tools to manage it, that our drive to self-medicate is on an entirely new level. Our great grandparents, no doubt, faced their own fear. Still, their stress was in the form of infrequent incidences (like a bad farming season), while our version of anxiety is frequent and emotional. We have financial, work, school, family, relationship, social, health, and other stresses accumulating at a seemingly constant rate. We are the most traumatized and stressed generation in human history, and our environment now allows us to escape, numb, and stimulate ourselves with unlimited access to unhealthy forms of self-medication. The combination of access to food and emotional turmoil is leading us to a critical mass of preventable diseases and conditions, like obesity.

Being Clear about Trauma

I have done my best to explain that trauma can stem from something as simple as having a parent who you feel doesn't understand or support you during times of emotional stress. But I fear that the stigma of trauma might make you think if you weren't physically or sexually abused you have not faced any trauma in your life. I believe this stems from a misunderstanding of the word itself. I don't say this to downplay severe injuries like abuse or to minimize the experiences of the people who have suffered them. In fact, I am hoping that making trauma more relatable to the average person will help us all to understand and empathize with the lifelong consequences of various forms of abuse.

It is now well known that trauma can begin in the womb. Children who are born to stressed mothers have a higher incidence of a variety of diseases and conditions. Asthma is a very well documented example. If you are born to a mother who faced an insurmountable degree of stress during her pregnancy, you have a markedly higher chance of developing asthma in your youth. The psychological state of your mother, even while you are still in the womb, is capable of changing your state of health.

Another example is children who are born to malnourished mothers. When infants are born underweight, they are much more likely to develop increased fat storage and grow into heavier children. It is hypothesized that the child is biologically prepared for a world of scarcity.

Trauma isn't isolated to childhood either. If you get into a car accident or witness someone get hit by a bus, there is the possibility you could develop a traumatic "wound" that leads you to the same set of problems that traumatic experiences can generate in earlier life. You aren't only susceptible to these issues in childhood, although you are much more vulnerable to them when you are young. This is commonly seen in PTSD often experienced by first-line workers who witness horrendous human death and suffering. This problem of adult trauma and the resulting PTSD is so severe that we are now facing a suicide epidemic in our first responders. I have close friends who are suffering the consequences of merely doing their jobs.

Trauma does not need to be thought of as a singular traumatic life event that happened when you were 8 years old. Your exposure to trauma began the day you were conceived and does not end until your life is over. From the cradle to the grave, so to speak.

The reason we are more susceptible to the effects of trauma when we are young is that we have fewer tools to deal with the events we face, and we are highly vulnerable to even the most minor forms of trauma. This is why parents are so closely connected to our adult "isms." Every tool or resource we lack when we are young is our parent's responsibility. A parent's primary role is to provide, teach, and protect when it comes to various stages in our growth. Think about the child who is being bullied at school who comes home to a father who says, "You just need to toughen up. Next time, punch him in the nose!" That child already feels scared, helpless, and like an outcast. He comes home to his protector and hears, "I am not here to support you. Take care of this matter yourself in the most terrifying way possible." That child is now left to cope with an incredible amount of stress, and the result will not be a positive one.

It is popular thinking today that we are a sensitive society, and we need to "toughen up." While I agree that outrage culture that inspires people to wear offence like a badge of honour is a problem, I wouldn't throw the baby out with the bathwater. When it comes to helping those we love to deal with issues they don't have the maturity, capacity, or resources to deal with on their own, I would say we need to increase our understanding and empathy. I also believe that those with the most aggressive "toughen up" attitudes were likely traumatized in their own lives. I am getting into the weeds a bit here, but it is essential to understand the emotional driving forces behind your most unhealthy behaviours.

Key Takeaways

· *Adverse life events result in unhealthy adult coping.*

· *It isn't about the scale; it is about your past.*

· *If you don't resolve emotional issues, it doesn't matter what you achieve. You will never feel good about yourself and constantly seek ineffective sources of wellbeing.*

· *These points are scientifically and clinically proven to be true.*

The more pain and suffering you faced in your past, the more you will seek self-medication in the present. What you continue to do in the future is entirely up to you. The worst kind of abuse often results in the most damaging forms of self-medication. More frequent and overlooked traumas (like bullying, social anxiety, and lack of support) are often self-medicated with food, alcohol, and technological distraction. If you can connect your present medication to your past suffering, you put yourself in a position to change your future.

CHAPTER 4: THE UNHEALTHY REWARD CYCLE

"[P]reaching at people about behaviours, even self-destructive ones, did little good when I didn't or couldn't help them with the emotional dynamics driving those behaviours."
— Gabor Maté, In the Realm of Hungry Ghosts: Close Encounters with Addiction

If you have read this far into the book, I congratulate you. Most people who seek answers for their weight problems are looking for a quick fix. That mentality rarely leads to a deep dive into the actual roots of health and fitness issues. I mention this because you should feel rewarded for your commitment to transforming your life. It is a good sign that this book isn't in your garbage can. It is typical (and understandable) to want to jump right into applying tactics to solve your problem. Still, as I mention throughout the book, you must comprehend the root of your self-harming behaviour if you are going to stop the downward spiral you are in.

In this chapter, you will be rewarded for your patience as we now begin to move toward your personal solution. So far, we have looked into our root issues very generally. We have been looking at the process of weight gain in the abstract. Getting specific will deepen your connection with your own root issues and help you apply successful long-term solutions for them. This process of deepening your relationship to your problems begins with what I like to call the unhealthy reward cycle.

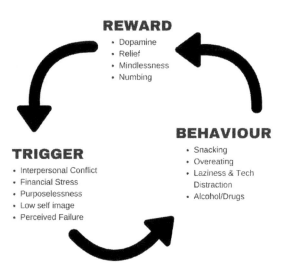

In the image above, you will see the basic process of what we have discussed thus far. The visual will help to show you how the operation of your mind can show up on your body. The material covered in this chapter will not be new to you, but now we can begin to clarify and organize what we've covered so far. Let's first break the image down.

The Trigger

Your unhealthy actions always begin with a trigger. These triggers vary by how sensitive we are to a given emotion or feeling. Anything from a fight with a loved one, to low finances, to feeling like you lack purpose can push you toward unhealthy self-medication. Here is a list of daily events, both big and small, that can act as the "trigger" that leads us into our most unhealthy behaviours.

Fighting with your spouse right before you go out the door to work
(Sensitivity to anger drives an emotional overwhelm that you numb with food at your desk at work)

Stepping on the scale in the morning and seeing it go up five pounds
(Sensitivity to sadness drives an emotional overwhelm that you stimulate your way out of with a sugary breakfast)

Getting a monotonous email from your boss saying he wants to speak first thing in the morning
(Sensitivity to fear drives an anxious rumination that you distract yourself from with chips and chocolate)

You look in the mirror after getting out of the shower, and you don't like what you see
(Sensitivity to self-disgust drives feelings of meager self-worth that you escape with alcohol and ice cream)

The list goes on and on. Triggers that lead to unhealthy behaviours do not need to be severe. Most of the time, we don't even recognize these thoughts and feelings as abnormal. We just chalk them up to being part of life. While these sorts of incidents make up a large part of our daily lives, the negative effect they can have on our future actions is much more profound than we think. I'm guessing as you read my short list, you could picture yourself in more than one of these emotional scenarios.

Severity

A trigger in isolation is rarely enough to hurt us. In fact, triggers that we can quickly deal with can often be extinguished, and therefore be a source of stress that disappears as soon as it came. Let's say you look into your savings account, and you have a negative balance. Worse, bills are going to come out of your account tomorrow. If you don't find some money, your mortgage will bounce. Sounds stressful. But if you have an investment account that you can quickly liquidate into cash, and you've got more than enough money in there to cover your balance, stress disappears. Or let's say you spill coffee all over yourself while trying to get into the car for work. If you have time to spare, you can go inside, change, and try again. If, however, you are already late, or worse, already at work and about to walk into an important meeting, your anxiety will be at level 10.

This is a bit of a simplification, but in general, the concept of severity stands. The severity of a trigger is dictated by your ability to deal with the stress it causes. In most of our lives, we are, in part, poorly equipped to extinguish many of our stressors in a healthy way.

The Behaviour

Now we get into the behaviour, the actions we take to avoid the pain of our emotional sensitivities. Common examples of these behaviours are overeating, late-night snacking, technological distraction, laziness, and alcohol consumption. Coping behaviour is as unique and differentiated as our personalities. As you know by now, these unhealthy behaviours are our attempt to self-medicate the adverse emotional effects of a stressor that we are not currently equipped to deal with. <I wold remove that sentence as the point has been made. As Dr. Mate would say, the behaviour is not the problem. Behaviour is an attempt to solve the problem. When assessing what is wrong with our lifestyle and what we need to change to get healthy and fit, these are the things we focus on. We don't realize that the behaviour is the end product of a trigger that could've happened eight hours ago. When we eat three bags of chips before bed, we rarely think "I really need to start going to bed earlier, so I stop rushing to work, spilling coffee all over myself and starting my day at level 10 stress and anxiety, thus resulting in endless late-night snacking." Instead, we think, "I need to stop eating junk at night." This disconnection from the driving force of unhealthy behaviours is the biggest reason why we rarely solve the problem in the long-term.

The Reward

The reward is what reinforces all of these poor behaviours and makes them stick. Worse, it helps them grow to be more powerful and more frequent. The reward is an extension of the dopamine cycle we discussed in the last chapter. Since you are familiar with the role of dopamine, I won't explain it again here. The reward is what drives the temporary relief we feel from the underlying stressor when we eat, drink, distract, and avoid. Many unhealthy actions result in psychologically favourable reactions like dopamine being released in the brain. When something like dopamine is released, we feel good in the short term. In the long run, we feel awful about our uncontrolled choice, which often leaves us emotionally worse off than we were before. In the moment, however, we are present bias. The stimulation, numbing, or distraction we receive from the unhealthy action in the moment blocks our ability to worry about what it will do to us in the future. Though we understand that eating cookies to avoid stress isn't serving us in the long run, rational thinking cannot be easily accessed in the present. Daniel Kahneman refers to this as system 1 vs. system 2 thinking. Hence the reason why these problems are easy to acknowledge after the fact, but rarely considered in the present.

To recap: We face an emotional stressor. If we are not equipped to resolve that stressor or if we are uniquely susceptible to that emotion, the severity of our drive to self medicate is increased. We self medicate with the most readily available sources of "painkillers." The temporary relief we get from these unhealthy actions reinforces their value in our brains. The demand for the drug grows as our dopamine reward system begins to dull. In the future, the mind will require higher dosages to provide the same amount of relief. This is how we get fat in a few years, even though we want nothing more than to be fit.

If you understand the unhealthy reward cycle, then you know how your surface-level behaviours get put into action. For many people, this is enough information on the subject. Others, however, will require an in-depth process to make these essential connections. That is why I created the 7 steps of manifestation. I thought about removing this chapter as I am risking being redundant. If you don't want additional information on this topic, please feel free to skip this section. If, on the other hand, you'd like to deepen your understanding of this process, please read on.

The 7 Steps of Manifestation

The unhealthy reward cycle acts as a basic explanation of *why* we get stuck in unhealthy coping behaviours. It is a quick way to reference what triggers and reinforces this problematic process. The 7 steps of manifestation will teach you what every potential step in the process looks like in your day-to-day life. Below I have provided an image to introduce you to this process.

TRIGGER
SENSITIVITY
OVERWHELM
INTENSIFIER
COPING
REINFORCEMENT
HANGOVER

As you can see, the steps that make up the unhealthy reward cycle are also present in the 7 steps of manifestation. A few details have been added. I find that this elaborated process is best introduced in story form. Seeing how these seven steps play out in a person's life will increase the likelihood that you can see them unfold in your own life as well. As I tell you the story of Jim, be sure to reflect on your own personal experience.

The story of Jim

It's Friday afternoon after a long week, and Jim can't wait for 4 o'clock to roll around so he can get out of the office. He's been in stressful meetings all week long and scrambling around the city in an attempt to tie up loose ends and hit his quarterly sales numbers. It's been a long week, but he has persevered. Jim survived another sales season and will be getting his much-needed bonus money. At the end of the day, he packs up his laptop to head out for the weekend. Then his boss walks in. "Jim, we need to talk about your performance this last quarter." Jim thinks to himself, "What is there to talk about?" Jim's boss explains that his last two big sales were not actually Jim's sales. The transactions that pushed him into bonus range were "split" sales between him and his coworker, Bob. Bob notified the boss that it was he who made the initial contact with the vendors on those sales. Although Jim did the final closing on the deals, it was Bob who initiated them. Standard practice in these scenarios is to split the sales tally between the two salespeople. As a result, Jim has failed to hit his quarterly goal, and the bonus he was so counting on will not be coming his way.

Jim was relying on that money to pay bills and get out of some debt that has been causing him significant stress. The bonus would've covered these expenses and given Jim some breathing room, but now what is he going to do? He also feels double-crossed by a coworker who is supposed to be his *friend.* That's two hard pills to swallow in a concentrated period.

The situation is not be the end of the world. However, Jim has struggled with success throughout his entire career. He came from a poor family with a lazy, unsuccessful father. Jim was embarrassed about his father and their financial troubles from a very young age. Jim was fired from his two previous jobs for underperforming, and as he gets older, he feels more and more like his father. Jim has developed a distaste for his father, so when he sees the similarity, Jim starts to develop an aversion to himself as well. This puts him in a troubled place.

Jim aims to resolve this trouble by heading to the local bar where he can see some familiar faces and blow off some steam. At the bar, he finds himself surrounded by overweight, surly, borderline alcoholics who are happy to indulge Jim's current frustrations. Jim feels like this environment is the only solution to his unbearable anxiety. He intends to have just a few drinks and a bite to eat. But two beers quickly turns into eight, and a "small bite to eat" turns into two plates of nachos, a rack of ribs, and two dozen wings. <Really that much? How about a plate of nachos, a rack of ribs and a dozen wings? The consumption of food and alcohol is numbing Jim. His problems seem to have disappeared from his mind, but he must keep up the act of consumption to stay numb.

The end of the night comes around, and Jim can't possibly eat or drink any more without risking a severe acute health problem. As the stimulation wears off, the emotional pain creeps back into Jim's head. During the cab ride home, all of his fears and anxieties come screaming back. Now he has the added regret of spending way too much money, and the self-medication has ultimately made him sick. He feels ashamed and guilty. He feels like a loser. Jim feels even more distraught and self-loathing than he did before arriving at the bar. Jim has gotten caught in the seven steps of manifestation. This is what most of us do in one form or another when faced with stressors we are not equipped to deal with properly. Let's look at where each one of these steps popped up in Jim's story.

The Trigger

Succumbing to an unhealthy action almost always begins with a painful trigger. This comes in the form of emotional pain and discomfort. A trigger could stem from a quarrel at work, a moment of low self-worth, or a high-stress personal situation (to name a few examples). The trigger is the first domino. For Jim, the trigger came in the form of acute financial stress and being wronged by a friend.

The Sensitivity

Your sensitivity to that pain is determined by adverse life experiences. Places in life where you have had emotional struggle will show up in the present when those wounds are touched again. Jim was embarrassed by his father's lack of financial success and likely grew up with feelings of insecurity and anxiety due to an unstable household. His current work situation brought him back to that place of embarrassment and fear.

The Emotional Overwhelm

When you are highly sensitive to a particular emotion, you become overwhelmed by it when it is triggered. As Jim's work situation unravels, he falls into a pit of anxiety and embarrassment. The emotional overwhelm grows beyond the possibility of an uncomplicated recovery.

The Intensifier

If Jim had significant sums of money in his bank account, or if he saw himself as a high performer who could quickly rectify his financial situation, he would get over this isolated incident. He would still be more sensitive to the emotions he felt as a result when compared to an individual without his history, but he would be able to move forward. But Jim is currently strapped for cash and behind on numerous bills. He doesn't have any financial or emotional support. This lack of tools and resources allows the emotional overwhelm to intensify.

The Coping

When we lack the right tools to progress from emotional overwhelm, we move to plan B. Unfortunately, plan B is a destructive form of escape. We eat until we are sick. We search out a sugar high. We drink. We sit on the couch in front of the T.V. for hours. We stay in bed for half the day. Jim went to the local bar and attempted to drown his anxieties with food and alcohol.

The Reinforcement

In the short term, Jim feels excellent. Perhaps more accurately, Jim doesn't feel much of anything at all. Chemical interactions in his brain respond positively to the excess of food and alcohol, which reinforces this sort of escape as an intervention. The problem is that our mind rarely accounts for the physical damage and emotional aftermath that follow these harmful actions.

The Hangover

In Jim's case, the hangover was literal. For most of us, the headache we experience after drowning emotionally in unhealthy self-medication is psychological. We feel guilty, ashamed, and often more anxious and unstable than we did before. This often lowers our self-image even more, and intensifies our emotional sensitivities. This pushes us deeper into the hole and completes the cycle.

The 7 Steps of Manifestation is a useful framework for summarizing what you now know. It is a breakdown of the events that connect your mind and waistline. Chances are your situation is not identical to Jim's. Still, it's easy to plug in your own unique struggles into this model. The last layer of this deep personal understanding of unhealthy behaviour is roots and reinforcements.

Behaviour, Root, and Reinforcements

When assessing our fitness issues, we tend to obsess over the big, unhealthy behaviours that we hold responsible for our poor health. We focus on uncontrollable overeating. We concentrate on snacking and late-night eating. We point the finger at Friday night pizza and wine traditions.

We tend to see these behaviours as the source of the problem. We think, "I am fat because I can't stop snacking at night." Our unhealthy actions no doubt result in issues like weight gain, but problems like overeating are just the surface level. By "surface-level," I am suggesting that these actions are not the root issues that need to be addressed. They are much more profound. There are clear patterns that lead to the unhealthy actions we take, and if you can recognize these patterns, you have a much better chance of shutting them down before they begin. Let's move to an example.

The Story of Nancy

Nancy has a problem with late-night snacking. She sees this

issue as the source of her weight gain. When she looks at herself in the mirror and sees her arms looking a little flabbier than just a few weeks ago, she blames it on her inability to cut out snacking. Nancy has steadily gained weight for the last 5 years. She has tried everything to kick the problematic habit but has not had any success. She has tried chewing gum to avoid cravings. She has tried sugar detox programs. Nancy has used every single ounce of her willpower to fend off the unrelenting need to eat at night, but she always succumbs. Sometimes she can go up to a week without giving in if she grits her teeth, but eventually, late-night snacking always wins.

Nancy has always assumed that she has some sort of genetic predisposition for sugar cravings. When 8 pm rolls around, her brain lets her know that it is time to snack. Nancy believes her mind has control over her, but as you will learn, it is actually Nancy who is telling her mind it is time to eat.

This is the typical late-night snacking pattern. Nancy gets home from a long day at work and begins preparing her dinner, which she sits down to eat at around 6:30 pm. After dinner, Nancy cleans up, doddles a bit, and thinks about what she is going to do that evening. Nancy *could* go for a walk or read a book, but those are daunting tasks at that time of night. She is tired and lacks the energy for anything remotely demanding. Without any other viable prospects to pass the time, Nancy heads to the couch and turns on her television. Time passes, and Nancy has watched 3 episodes of her latest Netflix binge. With the stimulation of the T.V. starting to fade, Nancy moves on to her laptop. Now she is scrolling through her social media networks with her television still running as background noise.

Then, just like clockwork, the craving sets in. Nancy resists, but after ten to fifteen minutes, she thinks to herself, "I'll just have one or two squares of that chocolate bar, no more than that." Nancy eats her first two chocolate squares. She fidgets. She tries to occupy her mind. But eventually, she goes back for a few more bites. Then she has a few more pieces. Then some popcorn. Then some chips. Before Nancy even realizes it, she is sucked into a food and technology-filled vortex. She is left feeling bloated and ashamed. She thinks to herself, "You weak idiot. This is why you are fat. You have no self-control."

What do *you* think is going on here? Has Nancy simply succumbed to an unhealthy snacking problem set off my her brain? Is this an issue of lack of willpower or weakness of character? That is what we usually believe when the dust settles after a binge. But here is what I have learned. The problem is not Nancy's lack of self-control. The problem is that Nancy has created a nightly routine that is ultimately going to end in a binge. It is Nancy's behavioural pattern that drives the eventual over-eating. This is how Nancy sees the problem: "I get a craving. I try to fight that craving. I lose the fight because I am weaker than my desires. The only solution is to focus on strengthened willpower."

With what you have learned so far, would you agree with Nancy's analysis? If not, what do you think is going on?

Dissecting Nancy's Snacking

If we trace back Nancy's steps, what do we find? Right before succumbing to the first craving for a few squares of chocolate, Nancy was mindlessly scrolling through social networks. Before that, she was lost in her T.V. shows. Before the T.V. was turned on, she was slowly sinking into the couch. And right before she decided to sit on the couch, she was talking herself out of doing something more productive like walking or reading. Do you see what is happening here?

Nancy's eating issues are not triggered by her craving mind. The craving does not exist on an island. Her idle mind, sterile environment, and lack of healthy stimulation are what lead Nancy into snacking mode. Sitting on the couch, turning on the T.V., and mindlessly scrolling through social networks have created the space for discomfort to set in. Nancy is now vulnerable to stress, boredom, and any other pain that she will undoubtedly attempt to escape. Boredom and lack of stimulation create the groove that Nancy has reinforced over time. This process began the moment she decided to sit on the couch instead of doing something productive. This is the root habit in the chain. Sitting down and "relaxing" is the beginning of the end for Nancy, and if her butt hits the couch after dinner, she is going to binge. The sofa is predictably followed by turning on the T.V., and eventually, the laptop. While Nancy mindlessly gets lost in gossip, her brain knows food is near. Her mind thinks, "Nancy is losing stimulation. I don't like this, I want some dopamine." Then, like clockwork, Nancy gets the signal to eat. Eating will temporarily extinguish the discomfort of boredom that is created and reinforced by this routine. Nancy feels good for now, and so does her brain. Her brain takes note of this routine and will only ask for greater stimulation in the future.

The behaviour, the craving, and the act of eating is not the problem. This is what we recognize as the problem (and therefore, where we put our behaviour change efforts). But this is inaccurate. In Nancy's case, lack of productivity and evening mindlessness constitute the problem worth solving. There are always signs that the behaviour is coming, but these subtleties are often ignored.

If the couch, the T.V., or the laptop were removed from the equation, the problematic surface behaviour (snacking) could be effectively modified.

And what about Nancy's reinforcing behaviours? Reinforcements are the actions or environment that exist alongside the problematic behaviours that allow them to thrive. In Nancy's case, she knows she has an issue with eating chocolate and chips. She knows that even at her most determined, she succumbs to out of control snacking. So why are there even chocolate and chips in her house to begin with? As most of us tend to do, Nancy justifies keeping the problematic food around. She'll say something like, "Oh, that isn't for me. I just keep it around for my nieces when they visit." Nancy probably also goes to the grocery store without a list of what she needs. If Nancy took some time to make a shopping list before going to the store, she would be less likely to justify buying junk. When she goes out and "wings it," it is much easier to grab a few snack foods without thinking about where they will end up. These are what are known as classic reinforcing actions, the things we do that allow us continued access to our big unhealthy behaviours. Following are some other examples of reinforcing behaviours.

· Hanging on to a McDonald's gift card you refuse to throw away. Next time you're in a morning rush, where do you think you'll stop to eat?

· Never having your workout and shower gear with you in the car so you can stop at the gym on the way home if you have some spare time.

· Going to a restaurant without looking at the menu ahead of time and selecting reasonable options.

·   Going to work hungry and/or empty-handed on a day when Pizza is typically brought in for lunch.

In these scenarios, you blame your hunger, lack of time, or lack of willpower for the outcome. In reality, you have unconsciously set yourself up for failure. You have allowed for an unsuccessful environment. It doesn't matter if we are talking about the big unhealthy behaviours or the habits and environments that support them. If you are falling into these cycles of harmful self-medication, you are doing so with a degree of mindlessness and a routine that lets your brain know the medication is coming. Strategies like eating less, cutting out snacking, and no more red wine at night never work in the long run for this reason. It is everything around the behaviour that needs to change.

Summing it all up

We have covered a lot of information thus far. Before moving on to the next section of the book where we will begin to solve behaviour problems, I want to summarize key takeaways.

The Evolutionary Barriers

These are the very *human* maladaptations that once served us well in the past, but in our modern environment are making us sick. They are the underlying drivers that are difficult to shut off because they were once (and in many ways, still are) necessary for our survival.

Key Takeaway: Being healthy is abnormal. Your current state of health is a human issue. It is not a matter of your

individual character.
Stress, Trauma, and Social Toxicity

These are the contemporary issues that are unique to today's human life. As human beings, we face past trauma, real-time stress, and societal toxicity that turn our once useful evolutionary instincts against our health. These modern problems play into our evolutionary barriers for maximized health struggles.

Key Takeaway: While the life of the modern human being is highly comfortable, it is also highly stressful. Adverse life experiences, daily stress, and social and emotional turmoil push us to self-medicate. This medication is powerful and abundant.

The Unhealthy Reward Cycle

You have a trigger (like stress) that is worsened by a lack of internal resources. The resulting discomfort pushes you into unhealthy coping behaviours. The harmful self-medication is reinforced by chemical reactions in the brain that are tightly linked to survival mechanisms. This reinforces food, alcohol, laziness, and technological distraction as an effective means of escaping the pain.

Key Takeaway: There is a process behind your most unhealthy behaviours. They are not random.

The 7 Steps of Manifestation

This is an in-depth model of the basic reward cycle to help you work out how unhealthy behaviours come to exist in your own life.

Behaviour, Roots, and Reinforcements

This is the surface level stuff that has created space for your most damaging behaviours. The content before this section detailed the underlying, universal drivers that subconsciously push all humans to be unhealthy. The response, roots, and reinforcements section shines a light on our surface-level actions.

Key Takeaway: Focusing on changing just the unhealthy behaviour always fails. You need to consider modifying everything that surrounds the response to improve the end product.

Part One of this book is now complete. I hope that you better understand the source of your worst health behaviours. In the next section of the book, we can begin your preparation for change by creating a platform for success. This is the only way to create sustainable health outcomes.

Key Takeaways

· *Sensitivity equals emotional suffering which equals self-medication.*
· *Modern triggers in sensitive emotional places end in unhealthy behaviours.*
· *Bad habits come quickly because the reward is immediate. Good habits come slowly because the reward is always delayed.*
· *You can train your system 2. You don't need to*

be a slave to system 1, but it takes time.

It doesn't take much to end up with three empty chip bags and a stomach ache. A fight with a loved one, a stressful commute, or even a poorly timed Instagram post can all drive you to self-medicate your emotional woes. Places where we are more likely to be emotionally sensitive drive unhealthy behaviours the most frequently. We usually self-medicate when we are mindless and disconnected from our emotional pain. We unconsciously trade our future health for immediate gratification. Understanding this process will help you recognize when it is happening. If you can see when it is happening, you can modify the outcome.

CHAPTER 5- ARE YOU READY TO CHANGE?

"When people are ready to, they change. They never do it before then, and sometimes they die before they get around to it. You can't make them change if they don't want to, just like when they do want to, you can't stop them."

— Andy Warhol (Andy Warhol in His Own Words)

When you picked up this book, you were motivated to take control of your health. Otherwise, you would've walked right past it. Perhaps, on the morning of your purchase, you sat down for breakfast, wearing a particularly tight pair of jeans. When you went to sit down, an uncomfortable roll of belly fat may have found its way overtop of your waistband. Or perhaps one of your parents recently commented on your body or choice of clothing in a hurtful way. Regardless of what motivated you to pick up this book, I want to be clear about something: motivation, inspiration, or whatever nudged you to buy this book is not sufficient enough to mark you as "ready" to apply my instructions. Wanting to change is very different from being prepared to change. If you are just at the wanting stage but not genuinely prepared, you will fail.

Inspiration and motivation can be a great way to kickstart your success. But many times, we put the cart before the horse and throw solutions at ourselves without first laying the proper groundwork. Inspiration can get the ball rolling, but it isn't enough to keep you in the game when the going gets tough, and trust me, the going *will* get tough. I'm not suggesting you should not act when you feel motivated. I am highlighting that taking action without being prepared is a big reason why inspired people end up failing in their first month of a fitness journey. You are probably telling yourself that this won't happen to you, but you would be naive to assume that you are any different than the general population. Based on the average statistical chance of failure (loosely, 95%), we should all understand that if we are not correctly set up for success, we will fail. I don't want to see that happen to you for the fifteenth time, and for that reason, I wrote this critical section on being prepared for change.

Many of you will hear a little voice in the back of your head right now that is begging you to skip this section and get to the action steps. Right now, the voice is saying, "You don't need someone to tell you whether you're ready or not. Just skip to the solution so you can start losing weight right now"! I would be surprised if this were the first time this little voice lead you astray. Although I cannot control you (or the little person in your head), I encourage you to take this piece of the process very seriously. Without understanding and applying the preparation tactics of this section, you may very well end up in the same place you have so many times in the past, frustrated and unsuccessful.

Think of the following preparedness work as the scaffolding needed to support your breakthrough. Without preparation, your dietary techniques have no support. If you don't have some solid objects to hammer your drywall into, how will it hang? Jumping into action without establishing your readiness will cause you the same problem you've always had. You will be desperately rushing toward a solution that you are not fundamentally prepared to put into action. You will be doomed to fall flat.

What it means to be "ready"

Most people don't understand the difference between "want to" and "ready to," and this is why most of us can't go 30 days before giving up on our weight loss efforts. *Wanting* to do something means that you have the desire to achieve a particular result. You want to be fit and healthy. Being *ready* to do something, on the other hand, is being *committed* to doing the necessary work to achieve the desired result regardless of your rate of success. The person who is "ready" is willing to sacrifice and do the work without any immediate proof of a result. You must assess where you see yourself on the readiness scale as you read through this section, because your level of readiness will determine what actions are reasonable for you right now. You probably think you fall into the "ready" bucket, but I encourage you to be open to changing that opinion. In this section, I aim to teach you the difference between "want to" and "ready to" and show you how to get yourself ready for a change. Doing so will increase the chances of lasting success.

The Fear of being Vulnerable is the Enemy of Readiness

Being "ready" is not about convincing yourself that you want something badly enough. It's easy to desire something and believe you can achieve it when you aren't in the thick of the challenges that are to come. Being ready is about allowing yourself to be vulnerable and being O.K. with that vulnerability. Are you comfortable with giving this mission everything you have and trying your best day in and day out, even if you fail miserably? Will you take the padding off of your ego and put it directly into harm's way for a shot at reaching your goal? Can you be honest about your weaknesses and shortcomings? Most of us cannot. We are not O.K. with being exposed. Transformation requires that you commit to taking healthy actions every single day no matter what happens (or doesn't happen) when you step on the scale and look for proof. It is exposing, and there is not a moment more painful than when you give a task everything you have, and you still don't succeed. At that moment, it's as though you prove to yourself that you are every awful name you've been calling yourself for the past decade.

For this reason, most of us don't try all that hard. We have spent so much of our lives building up defence systems and blockades between ourselves and potential hurt that we can't see that we are sabotaging our chances at success, health, and happiness. We can't see the escape routes we leave open for our ego. If we never *really* try, we can save face when we give up and fail on our goals. More on that later. For now, let's take a closer look at why we aren't prepared for change: we want to avoid being vulnerable.

When goals are very personal, like those that involve our body, we are particularly afraid of trying. We go through life building walls each time we face pain, adversity, or disappointment. This way, when we face a similar scenario in the future, it doesn't hurt as bad as it did the first time. Tough skin is not a positive trait, because thick skin doesn't just prevent the hurt from penetrating our mind. It also prevents success from entering our lives.

Because of this, we tend to set little escape routes that we can squeeze through when we feel like failure is on the horizon. We do this to soften the blow, and we accomplish it through a wealth of lies. So what form do these escape routes take? How do you know if you are not vulnerable enough to change?

Here is a non-fitness example to which most of us can relate. What happens when you give yourself to a man or a woman only to have your heart trampled on? When you are open to love, you are vulnerable. What if shortly after falling for that person you find out you weren't the only one or that the person never loved you the way you loved him or her? You walk away from that relationship so hurt that you build internal defence systems that prevent you from being hurt again in the future. You become closed, resentful of relationships, and you begin to devalue the role of a significant other. Many of us spin these sorts of defence mechanisms as strength and independence, but putting walls up is the opposite of power. It is an example of pure fear. In this case, it is fear of giving someone your heart only to have it smashed into a million pieces. The surest way of preventing that pain in the future is never to put your heart in another person's hands. How does that fear affect your future relationships? It makes it nearly impossible to have meaningful ones. Your hardened skin prevents you from being hurt again, but at the cost of never being able to experience a successful relationship. You protect yourself from love by never allowing yourself to experience it. We do the same thing when we struggle with our health. When we dedicate ourselves to a diet and exercise program only to fall short of our goal, we feel like failures. We create a system of defence that prevents us from being vulnerable enough to suffer the same anguish in the future. But much like the relationship analogy, these defence systems also stop us from being vulnerable enough to let success in the door. Succeeding requires 100% effort and trust in what we are doing. Once we have felt the pain of failure, we have a habit of never genuinely giving ourselves to the transformation. That way, if we fail, we can always tell ourselves that we didn't give it everything we had. This is how we save face, and this is what prevents our readiness for change and future success.

In cognitive behavioural therapy, this is referred to as your "core beliefs" and "automatic thoughts." Core beliefs are the nasty little filters your thoughts go through that make you feel bad about yourself. These filters are created during the adverse life events that we covered earlier in the book. A verbally abusive parent, a socially awkward or unhealthy childhood, being bullied and made fun of, or comparing oneself to others are examples of ALE's(?) that lead to negative core belief systems. Let's look at core beliefs through the relationship example used earlier. If you've shown admiration for people in life only to have been rejected, you might begin to tell yourself that you are ugly, or fat, or dull. You must somehow make sense of the rejection. Facing too many of these incidences, or fewer if more , will create a negative filter for your future relationships and social interactions. You think less rationally and more defensively. If a date cancels on you, it can't be due to a family emergency or a work crisis; it's because he or she isn't attracted to you, or because you said something idiotic. This is where your mind automatically goes. In your health, the process is the same. Your feelings of being weak or lazy and not "deserving" to be healthy are examples of core beliefs. You reinforced these negative core beliefs each time you tried and failed to take control of your health. In the past, you let yourself be vulnerable when trying to get in shape. If you didn't reach your arbitrary measurement of success, you reinforced a belief system that used your worst assumptions about yourself to explain your lack of success. These beliefs likely started growing in your mind at a very young age.

Core beliefs can be either conscious or unconscious but mostly unconscious. And these primarily unconscious beliefs lead to harmful automatic thoughts. The example I used earlier of "this person canceled our date because s/he doesn't find me attractive" is an example. It is not the most likely explanation, but it is the explanation you choose when your core beliefs are self-defeating. Your feelings of being unworthy of love drive you to assume all situational outcomes stem from a negative place. Simple examples of these automatic thoughts in health would go something like "you can't stop eating chips because you're a fat, undeserving loser" or "you never exercise because you're weak and don't have the willpower that healthy people do." Those thoughts might sound incredibly nasty, but let's be honest, you are more offensive to yourself than anyone else you encounter in life will be to you. Core beliefs and automatic thoughts have been dictating your attitude toward your "self" for a long time, and with opinions and feelings like those, it's no surprise that you're terrified to give your body the love and effort it deserves. You have built such thick skin and emotional defences that now it has become impossible for you to succeed. You become paralyzed.

Fearful of having these beliefs and thoughts become reality (thus proving everything we think about ourselves), we establish escape routes. We lie to ourselves, and to others. Both lies are equally damaging. These protective lies we tell can be superficial or deep. Superficial lies are the ones we voice audibly, like not being honest to a coach about what you eat at night. Deep lies are the ones we only tell ourselves. Both superficial and deep lies can prevent us from succeeding, and since they stem from our core beliefs, they can be hard to kick. Here are some examples of these common forms of self-sabotage.

Superficial Lies

What we say

"I can dedicate myself and lose weight. No problem. I just need someone to tell me what to eat and what exercises to do."

The reality

If this is true, why are you still looking for help? If success were a matter of having information and guidance, you would have succeeded by now. It just hurts too badly to say, "I'm a mess. I eat until I'm sick to my stomach every night. I'm out of control." So instead, we pretend to have it all together, which prevents us from getting the help we need.

What we say

"It's my family. They are so unhealthy. My husband eats chips all night, and my kids eat sugary cereals and snacks. They're the reason why I keep failing."

The reality

While having a household that doesn't have the same values and goals as you certainly doesn't help, it isn't a valid excuse for failure either. Instead of looking at yourself as the source of your problems, you are externalizing your issues onto other people. If you can point the finger at someone else, you don't have to face the fact that you are the problem.

What we say
"I can do it, but I just want you to know that I'm not willing to give up my dark chocolate and red wine"!

The reality

First of all, if you were prepared to change, you would be willing to give up anything. The refusal to give up unhealthy food and drink is not you taking a stand. Setting strict boundaries that protect unhealthy habits as though it were a strength is just another way of saying "I don't have any confidence in turning my habits around."

Deep Lies

What we say
"You don't deserve this."
"You'll never be healthy. You're too darn lazy."
"Here you go, doing what you always do. You're such a screw-up."

The reality

We can analyze all deep lies in the same way. Taking our health back is something we value. We want it *so* badly. But we also lack the confidence to *believe* we can achieve it. Because of this, we tell ourselves these deep lies so that when we fail, we can see it as *expected.* If we expect failure, we won't be hurt as badly if and when we do fail. We are conditioned to be self-defeating, for if we defeat ourselves before we even try, we avoid the future pain of failure. For instance, if you start a new diet but go into it with refusal like "I'm not giving up my red wine and chocolate," you are protecting yourself. You are saying, "If I refuse to give up my red wine and chocolate, I can always use that refusal as my excuse for not reaching my goal." We use these deep lies to reinforce our defences so that if we fail, we aren't so hurt by it. If deep down, you tell yourself you are never going to succeed, failure is less painful. You'll know it was too good to be true right from the start.

The cruel joke in this process is that if we did away with the lies altogether, we would never fail. I know that sounds crazy, but it's true. If you let down our defences and allow yourself to be vulnerable, you can give a mission everything you have. You will be so resilient in the face of adversity that, over time, in spite of ups and downs, you will persist and reach your health goals. Once you start creating the escape routes with thoughts like "I'm not willing to give up chocolate" and "I'll never be able to keep this progress up, any day now that scale is going to move in the other direction" you have already set the course for disaster. You have created and dictated your own failure.

If you are going to change, you must first be O.K. with being fully vulnerable, much like how the person who has been hurt must get past the pain to love again. You must be willing to face tough times with strength and deal with poor choices without personal judgment. You must be willing to persist with healthy actions regardless of what the scale says. I call this attitude "health without strings attached." You have to be ready to leave all of your excuses behind and say, "this is on me, nobody else. If I fail, it's because I let my negative thoughts get the best of me, and if I fail, that's O.K. It doesn't say anything about me as a person, and it's just an opportunity to learn about myself and improve." That may sound like a tall order, and it is, but when you shut down your negative beliefs and automatic thoughts, you close the escape routes and avoid the lies that you up for failure. When you do this, you succeed, perhaps not in 6 months or even a year, but you will succeed. Be willing to give it everything you have, even if you could end up disappointed. Otherwise, you will never reach your goal and will continue wasting your life jumping from one diet to the next.

A Note about "Expectations"

One of the biggest mistakes I see people make during a transformation is setting expectations. To paraphrase a quote I read, "Setting expectations is making a promise to suffer in the future." That about sums it up.

People often want to lose a certain amount of pounds in a certain amount of time. They say, "I need to lose 25 pounds by the summer." Here is the problem with specific goal-based expectations: your body does not change on your predetermined timeline. This means there is little chance you will reach your expectations. It also means your chances of being disappointed and defeated are high. Most people need to focus on their trajectory, and action-based goals. Good is good. If you want to lose 25 pounds in six months, and you lose 11 instead, you might see that as a failure. How ridiculous is that? But this is how we see achievements when we have set expectations. If you are eating out eleven times per week, try to get that down to four or five times per week and measure that instead. If you get to the gym once every two weeks, get that up to two to three times per week and track that metric. Those are the expectations worth setting: the ones you can control.

Denial, False Realities, Enabler Seeking, and Normalization

Negative thought patterns are the main reason people aren't prepared for change, but other forms of self-sabotage arise once you begin your transformation journey. These are the lies we tell and the traps we set once we are already in the process of change. You must recognize them for what they are because they will creep into your head as you change your diet and exercise habits. The first form of self-sabotage is that of denial.

The Power of Denial

When we are about to self-sabotage our goals, we preempt the problematic behaviour with some form of denial. We do this to clear our conscience and avoid cognitive dissonance. Every time you eat food that you shouldn't, or you skip the gym; denial makes it easier for you to forget what you are trying to achieve. Denial comes in the form of rationalization, minimization, and making excuses. These self-sabotaging thoughts serve as a free pass to engage in unhealthy behaviour. Here are some examples using pizza. I use pizza because it is universally delicious, and I can't imagine anyone who couldn't place themselves in a situation where pizza may be tempting. If pizza doesn't tempt you, I'm not sure why you are reading this book.

In a typical scenario, your friend or significant other asks you if you want to order pizza for dinner. "That jerk," you think. "Doesn't s/he know I am trying to lose weight?" You understand that eating pizza is not going to get you any closer to your goals. Still, your lower brain is saying "cheese, bread, salt, calories...deliciousness! Eat that pizza!" So instead of suggesting something less destructive for dinner, you begin to construct denials that allow you to give in to your lower brain. We are masters at doing this while not registering the event as an unhealthy act. You are laying your escape routes that protect your ego from self-sabotaging actions. That is the background story, and here are the fundamental denials you might utilize in a situation like this.

Rationalization: "I worked hard this week, my body probably needs pizza because of all the exercise I've done. If I eat something with fewer calories, I won't properly recover from my workouts."

Minimization: "It's just dairy, protein, vegetables, and a tiny bit of bread. How is that not healthy food?"

Excuse-making: "Well, my friend wants pizza. How can I say no? He twisted my arm, and I don't want to be a dietary outcast."

Does any of this sound familiar?

When you redesign the situation favourably, it makes it easier for you to go against your better judgment. You end up taking part in unhealthy actions without the guilt. But we all know that guilt-free indulgences never remain guilt-free. Harmful self-justified actions will lower our self-worth and let us down internally. We must push back against denial. Being brutally honest and having the ability to recognize these defensive excuses is not easy work, but it is certainly necessary for success.

I'm not saying that if you're trying to lose weight and improve your health, you can never have a slice or two of pizza. You don't have to avoid every birthday party and social event that may include temptations and indulgences. I'm suggesting that when you use denial to filter your thinking, you are protecting yourself from the reality of the decision you are making. Refusal not only makes it easier to take part in unhealthy acts, it also makes it more likely that you will mindlessly overindulge. You have convinced yourself that the consequences of your deleterious action are small or non-existent. Being honest is what is most important. You can still indulge. Just be careful in how you frame the indulgence and picture how you'd prefer the indulgence to happen.

You need to frame it like "Don't make any excuses. Don't go down the path of denial. You know that eating pizza is not going to get you closer to your goals, and you are likely going to feel bad if you eat ½ a large pizza. Limit yourself to 2 slices, no more. Take your time, chew slowly, and enjoy each bite. After that, do your best to cease the pizza eating. If you eat more than a few slices, you'll just be abusing the food, not enjoying it."

Use the recognition of denial as an opportunity to create a mental landscape that moves you toward self-control. Otherwise, you will fall into the denial based thinking that leads to a loss of all control. We will go into specific techniques in this area in future chapters, but for now, I want to continue on this path by talking about the issue of false realities.

False Realities

Another common problem fallible human beings face is the inability to live in reality. Psychological mechanisms known as heuristics and biases trick us into seeing our lives through rose-colored glasses. It is easy to paint a picture of living the perfect, healthy life while blaming failure on genetics, bad advice, or age. We opt to remember history in a way that favours our ego. If we create memories where our lack of success is someone else's fault, it hurts less when we look at our bellies. This inaccurate reflection is another example of the lies we tell ourselves to protect our ego from anticipated failure. For instance, human beings are notoriously poor calorie counters. Some studies suggest we consume twice as many calories as we estimate. We forget the frequent bites, the cream in our coffee, and the excessive dressing on our salad. Or we just flat-out lie about it. In either case, the result is the same. We think to ourselves, "I've only been eating 1400 calories per day, I should be losing weight!" This is easy to say when we conveniently ignore a thousand calories we consumed through nibbles and bites. We also grossly overestimate how many calories we burn through exercise and remember ourselves as being far more active than we are. We ignore our weekend bender of alcohol and dinners out when retroactively assessing our past week's behaviours. We think, "I don't get it. I stuck to my diet, went to the gym, and did all of the right things last week, but I'm up 3 pounds. This is so frustrating. Nothing works for me!"

These patterns of thought result in false recollections that make it hard to adjust what we are doing to continue progressing. This is why honesty and facts are so important. If you're lying to yourself about what goes into your body (as well as how often you are moving it), you can't be a good judge of what you might need to change in your plan. Diet and exercise don't work for the pretend person you recall in your head. The *actual* you who added on an extra 600 calories per day in bites, nibbles, and neglected food toppings is the person who needs to be assessed. How quickly we forget about mindlessly eat at night, the hours spent on the couch, our consumption of wine or beer, and the fact that we are eating at a drive-thru on the way to work each morning. It is easier to lie and deceive than it is to be brutally honest. We are willing to sacrifice our health in exchange for not taking responsibility for our actions, and it means most of us struggle to take our health back.

Incorrect assumptions are just another form of self-protection. They are natural, human, and understandable. You are not unique in this scenario. But that doesn't mean working on removing the lies from your self-defensive approach to fitness isn't your responsibility to fix. If we can convince ourselves and others that we are doing everything correctly, we can justify quitting. Blaming our lack of health on a non-existent genetic disorder, or the diet and exercise method we used that has failed us, becomes our default excuse. Deception blocks your success, so cut it out.

Enabler Support

Who doesn't love the friend who rushes over when you are cracking a bottle of wine and opening up a box of pizza after a long week at work? Even better is their telling you you look great and they don't understand why you are trying to stay on a diet. "You know, it's probably not even good for you to be cutting back on food. You eat like a rabbit. I don't even know how you're surviving." This is the sort of stuff we secretly love to hear as it allows us to give in to the stimulating behaviours that move us away from our goals. Picture your "friend" encouraging you to break your diet with a mouthful of pizza, a 16 oz glass of wine, and 50 pounds to lose on their waistline. This is your favourite type of friend, far better than the one who would show up and tell you that a bad week at work isn't a justification for eating and drinking your pain away.

There's a reason why we don't like to spend time with people who tell us the truth. They reveal to us the reality of our poor choices, and as we know, our ego and defence systems do not like what reality has to offer. If we had more truth-tellers in our lives, we would make far fewer poor food decisions. But in our toxic culture, it is considered normal to indulge regularly and be overweight and sick. It is abnormal to be conscious of one's health and act accordingly, so surrounding ourselves with truth-tellers is rare. In our society, people don't make friends by reminding each other of their mistakes, even though these are precisely the type of relationships we should value most. We don't want our friends and family members pointing out that we complain about our weight out of one side of our mouth while shovelling potato chips into the other. We don't appreciate reminders of our inconsistencies and lies.

For this reason, we tend to gravitate to those who we know will play along with us. When we are feeling down and discouraged, we don't call the friend who is going to tell us, "It's your fault, suck it up, and stop feeling sorry for yourself." We are going to call the friend that says, "it's O.K., it's not your fault, you're only human, let's meet and talk about it over a cheeseburger." This approach works out well for both parties because the enablers we seek are coincidentally also the people who subconsciously wanted us to fail. Most facilitators aren't intentionally sinister. Still, many people who love us don't want to see us succeed in an area where they feel weak. If you look at your peer group, they are likely suffering in many of the same ways you are, so they have the same negative core beliefs and fears that you do. When we take steps to change our health, it is threatening to those around us who are insecure and wish they could also improve their health but don't believe that they can. If you begin to get fitter and healthier, how is that going to make your unhealthy friends feel? Not too good. Your progress is a threat to their egos. Enablers are the people in our lives who pressure us to eat and drink foods and beverages that we already said "no" to five times. They are the people who aim to make us feel like outcasts for ordering a salad instead of a baked potato. These are the people who have put the spotlight on us for having only one glass of wine while they drink themselves into a stupor. "What are you, on a diet or something"? Luckily for this group, we often succumb to the pressure and give in to their unhealthy suggestions. It's the perfect relationship. We get permission to act in a way that is contradictory to our goals, and they get to feel better about the actions they aren't taking.

It is important to note that this enabler relationship is the opposite of compassion, while the approach that a truth-teller would take is the epitome of kindness and compassion. This is an important distinction to make because jealousy and insecurity are often passed off as being caring. Compassion is not lying to someone about his or her reality, so they can continue to live in an unrealistic world. That is cruel and unhelpful. Compassion means helping someone you love to establish the truth about their current reality, without judgment, so they can begin to thrive. If you looked at your child's report card and read he is violent with other kids, rude to teachers, and destructive of school property, how would you feel? Would you gently stroke your child and say, "Oh, it's not your fault, you're a good boy, those teachers just don't know what they are talking about"? This would set your child down a destructive path, never addressing whatever internal pain led to this extreme acting out. Is that care and compassion for your child? Kindness cannot live outside reality.

I'm not saying that you need to ditch your friends and family members to be healthy (although there *are* occasions where this may be warranted). Support plays a huge role in success, and you need relationships to have help, but you need to ask yourself what type of support you're getting from those around you. You need to be aware of your tendency to look for help when you should be looking for a reality check. Some people in your life are going to happily drag you down out of fear that you will outgrow them in some way. You know what you are going to get from the peer group who thinks your attempts to be healthy, happy, and confident are, in some way, a problem. Just like the alcoholic who can't keep himself away from the old gang at the bar, you will often gravitate toward the people who reinforce your unhealthy coping rather those who remind you when you are compromising your health and goals. You might not be able to control the number of enablers in your life — For some of us, the worst ones are our husbands, wives, and significant others — but you *can* control your habit of looking to them to absolve your health sins. Be aware of your tendency to seek out enabler support instead of dealing with the reality of your unhealthy actions. Owning up to your harmful activities can be helpful, if not liberating, if you look at it through the correct lens.

Normalization

The last piece of the preparation puzzle relates to our tendency to normalize unhealthy behaviours and allow societal norms to support our self-sabotage. I left this for the end of the chapter because it contains a little bit of everything we've covered thus far. An example of normalization would be: "Food is a social thing, and human beings are designed to connect over food and drink, so it's weird to go to a party and not eat the dips and drink the alcohol." The driving force of normalization is the toxic culture that is western society. While it's true that human beings *are* social eaters, that has little to do with the foods we choose to put into our bodies. You can be social with healthy eating and reasonable beverage choices- not just pizza, beer, and cake. We are normalizing unhealthy actions on a personal, cultural, and societal level to justify harmful actions while ignoring the internal voice that tells us eating until we are sick is a bad idea. We give in to the cravings that distract us from the woes of modern human life, and it is killing us in record numbers.

Societal normalization and the acceptance of unhealthy lifestyles have gotten so abundant that it is incredibly rare not to be overweight. Almost one half of us are obese, and even more of us are at least overweight. Those numbers should be making your head spin. If I were to tell you that 50% of us had type 1 diabetes and 70% of us had type 2 diabetes, I think you'd be appropriately shocked. But in the case of overweight, there is no shock because it has become so commonplace.

Our society supports, encourages, and perpetuates consuming fast food and sugary drinks, drinking socially, being minimally active, and adopting the myriad "isms" that constitute being a modern human. Most members of contemporary society have such abundance that we don't even know what it feels like to be hungry.

It is easy to let yourself fall back into old habits when the most unhealthy of us make up the majority. Less than one in three of us will get through adulthood without suffering some preventable lifestyle-driven disease. Being sick isn't healthy, but it is shockingly common.

Summary

It is one thing to be inspired to change, but it is quite another to be ready to change. If you aren't prepared for change, your chances of success are slim. I am willing to bet that any person who attempts to take control of their health without honestly facing the internal issues we have covered in this chapter isn't going to have a chance of succeeding. That doesn't mean that you need to be perfect to begin your transformation. It just means that you need to be aware of your unhelpful defences, your common signs of denial, false realities, enabler seeking, and the societal normalization that helps you sweep your worst behaviours under the rug. You will hit bumps in the road along the way. You will face setbacks that are emotionally challenging. You will slip up. You will gain weight. You will do many of the things you know you aren't supposed to do while trying to improve your health. This is all part of what it means to be a success story.

The difference between the person who succeeds and the person who fails is simple. The person who succeeds lives in reality, and the person who fails fears reality. The successful person also reflects on their mistakes without judgment. Doing so allows you to implement strategies for improvement and keep moving forward. Persistence is the name of the game. The person who fails is so closed, dishonest, and fragile that the slightest hiccup in the journey will result in such deep hurt that it becomes easier to never really try. The more you understand the escape routes you set for yourself and your internal defence mechanisms, the better chance you have of dealing with them positively. You need to be self-aware and stop blaming every indulgence you make on your character. The person who can make a mistake, forgive themselves, and move on is the person who will inevitably succeed. The person who makes every slip-up personal can never persist in the face of a daily emotional beating.

Key Takeaways

- *Wanting to change is not the same as being ready to make the sacrifice necessary to progress*
- *You will look to others to support your way of life, even though you know it is hurting you*
- *If you act without preparation, you will fail, 100% of the time*
- *You will constantly fool yourself into thinking your unhealthy actions are warranted*

Everyone wants better health. Everyone would also like to have more money, better relationships, and a 100-foot yacht. The trouble is that craving is the easy part. Being in a position to apply the necessary actions for change requires more significant consideration. Sometimes it is good to move quickly toward a goal, but only if you are genuinely prepared to do what is necessary to get results. Otherwise, you will end up frustrated and defeated.

CHAPTER 6-THE MYTH OF MOTIVATION

"It is when we act freely, for the sake of the action itself rather than for ulterior motives, that we learn to become more than what we were. When we choose a goal and invest ourselves in it to the limits of concentration, whatever we do will be enjoyable. And once we have tasted this joy, we will redouble our efforts to taste it again. This is the way the self grows."

— Mihaly Csikszentmihalyi, Flow: The Psychology of Optimal Experience

Mihaly Csikszentmihalyi is the acclaimed author of the "Flow" book series. He is also a man I have had the privilege of speaking with on multiple occasions regarding the work that I do. Mihaly has spent decades trying to understand the roots of happiness and success. He is the world leader in this area of study. "Flow" is the term he coined for the state of effortless productivity and the "loss of time" that a person experiences while they are performing a meaningful task. Picture the musician who plays with such fluency that her instrument seems to be an extension of her body. Or consider the gymnast who is so connected to his movement that he makes the world his endless playground. These people are experiencing "flow" when their minds and bodies complete complex tasks with seemingly minimal effort. In his book, Mihaly discusses how these extraordinary people have become so successful in their area of expertise. He refers to the specific act of practice without needing anything in return as being "autotelic."

Autotelic means having within itself its own purpose. It is doing something for the intrinsic reward, without attachment to a specific outcome. For example, Bill Gates succeeded in the world of computers because he was obsessed with emerging technology. He put in long nights, had a lot of luck, and got into the industry at just about the perfect time, but that wasn't the catalyst for his success. If Bill Gates didn't become a multi-billionaire in the world of technology, he would likely still be in a basement somewhere messing around with computers. *That is why* Bill Gates succeeded. He was truly fascinated and invested in what he was doing. It was the reward and satisfaction of the day to day experience and experimentation that drove him, not a desire to be the richest man on the planet. If Bill Gates were trying to be the richest man in the world, chances are he wouldn't have amounted to much. We see musicians like Adele performing moving songs in front of massive crowds and we forget that she has spent the majority of her musical career in a small room somewhere, playing the piano for hours on end. No fans, no payment. Just countless hours of practice for the sake of improvement. We see the product of her ultimate success and forget that success didn't drive her to superstardom. The love of music that kept her glued to her piano is what led to her success. It was not the desire to be a famous musician.

So what do Bill Gates, Adele, and Mihaly have to do with your ability to lose weight and be healthy? The answer is "a lot." When you are starting your weight loss journey, what is your motivating factor? You likely had a moment of low self-image that lead to setting an arbitrary, time-based goal. For example: "I look and feel disgusting. I need to lose 30 pounds by February. That will make me feel better about myself." That is the typical formula that we use to drive change: a moment of negative emotion followed by a random physical goal, that if reached, will permit you to feel like a person of value. You are looking to the result to provide satisfaction rather than the act of taking care of yourself. Focusing on the result is a big mistake, and it is one of the main reasons why people fall off of the wagon when trying to take control of their health.

Here's why. You are setting an expectation that gives you little control over the outcome, thus guaranteeing a future of disappointment and failure. Let's say you set a goal to lose 30 pounds in three months. You will likely pick this goal because results in a weight that takes you to a time when you felt better about your body. You probably picked the three-month timeframe because you have an event coming at that time, or because you know someone who lost that amount of weight in that timespan, therefore you should be able to do it too. We base our goals on random external benchmarks. Whatever got you to this specific goal and timeline, it wasn't the result of well thought out calculations. It was purely an emotional equation. That may seem inconsequential, but what happens when you are two months into your efforts, and you've only lost eight pounds? You are going to feel like a failure. You set a goal, you made an effort, and with thirty days left, you are sure to miss your target. The likely human response is to say some nasty things to yourself and stop the effort. But wait a minute - didn't you lose eight pounds? Isn't that a good thing? You'd think so, but your arbitrary goal with a timeline has prevented you from celebrating your success. So an eight-pound weight loss may as well have been an eight-pound weight gain. You may be wondering where I am going with this. We are told so often how important it is to have specific and measurable goals. Now I am telling you that having particular, quantifiable goals is a mistake? What gives? The goal is not the issue. The issue is how we frame the goal.

Trajectory + Action > Goals

Everyone needs a goal, but who says goals need to revolve around a scale, clothing size, or measurement? What you need is a trajectory with specific actions that will keep you on that trajectory. For instance, if I were to ask you what you needed to do to lose weight, you might respond with something like, "stop snacking at night, go to the gym more, and eat better meals." What if I asked you to dig a little deeper and tell me what you need to do to achieve those ends? You might say, "I would need to spend more time making my own meals, I'd need to go to the gym first thing in the morning, and I would need to watch less T.V. because that is when I mindlessly snack." Perfect. Now turn what you just said into your measurable goals. Example: I need to make my own dinner at least five nights per week. I need to get up at 5:30 AM three times per week and have my gym gear ready so that I can get my exercise in. And I need to limit my T.V. watching to one hour per night, which will also help me get to bed before 11 PM." There you go, you have your goals worth measuring. There is also a place for your superficial measurements of success, be it the scale, clothing size, or however else you objectively measure how you are doing. But external measurements should be done less frequently, and you should look at them through the lens of trajectory, not specificity. For example, if you want to use the scale, go for it, but only weigh yourself once or twice per month, and if your weight is moving in the direction you want it to move, that is a success, and you should feel good about it. If the scale isn't moving in the right direction, you evaluate and adjust your measurable actions.

But what about people who set specific goals and achieve them? We all know someone who set a goal to lose a certain amount of weight and was able to do so. And we've all seen a wealth of weight-loss success stories on the internet; so how can I say that specific, time-based goals are ineffective? My first answer is that there will always be outliers. There will always be a small percentage of the population who succeed within a structure that would lead most others to failure. But looking for lessons in exceptions is a mistake. My second answer is that anyone can grind it out for a few months, suffer, and achieve a goal that they cannot sustain. The willingness to suffer in the short term to attain a quick goal is what I call "grinding it out" in fitness. Any extreme weight loss protocol can produce success stories that last thirty or sixty days, sometimes even a year. What these methods don't have, however, is the ability to deliver long term results. If you tell someone they can lose 30 pounds in 30 days by drinking low calorie shakes, thus creating a massive energy deficit (much like the Isagenix "cleanse" model), most people will be able to grind it out and lose quite a bit of weight. This is not a surprise. In the world of psychology, it is well-established that human beings can mentally and physically handle scenarios they know are temporary. This is why most people can tolerate extreme short term dietary interventions. If you tell a man he needs to live in a jail cell for 14 days, he can do so with minimal suffering because he knows when the confinement will end. If, however, you stick a man in a jail cell and tell him that he will remain there from 24 hours to 24 years (even though you will release him after 14 days), he will suffer extreme mental anguish in those two weeks. The popularity of 30-day challenges, 14-day cleanses, and other such regimens is as high as it is for that reason. People want results, they want them now, and they can suffer for a short term period to get them. People just can't keep them.

Any result you obtain by using a particular strategy will not endure if you stop following the approach that got you there. The weight you lose on a 30 day "cleanse" will only stay off your waistline if you live the rest of your life on low calorie shakes or whatever extreme protocol got you the initial weight loss. If you want to keep results or continue improving in the future, you must be able to sustain the daily actions it took to achieve the progress in the first place. People can't do this, so they fail. It may take a month, six months, or a year, but you can bet failure is on the horizon. "Fitness hygiene" as I like to call it is just like dental hygiene. You can't brush your teeth one month out of every year and expect great dental health year-round. The same goes for your fitness. Whatever actions you take each day to improve your fitness must remain as part of your regular lifestyle if you are to retain those benefits.

So what do these points have to do with Mihaly's "flow" principle and your weight?. **If you want to succeed in your health and fitness goals, you must take an autotelic approach**. You must find ways to better your health that you would continue to work on and apply to your life *regardless* of the cosmetic result. Remember that Bill Gates and Adele each reached massive success not because they could see fame and riches in their future, but because they integrated daily practice that was self-fulfilling. The result was a by-product of the practice. You, too, will reach success not by obsessing over a waistline size or number on the scale, but by integrating healthy actions that you value and enjoy. Taking daily steps that move you toward a superficial result, but cause you to suffer, will never be sustainable. I am not suggesting that you shouldn't have any cosmetic health goals. We all have our vanity, and weight loss *does* mean (in most cases) better health, so losing weight is not that superficial a goal. If you force yourself to achieve those goals through daily actions that are not self-fulfilling, you will never succeed in the long run. We have a habit of making extreme initial sacrifices to lose weight quickly instead of focusing on finding the joy in taking care of ourselves. It is the joyful actions that build fitness discipline over time. And control is what makes healthy habits stick. So if you want to implement a healthy daily routine that will lead to long-term success in your health, you must find alternative motivations for healthy actions. I will use the rest of this chapter to teach you how you can make this happen.

Do What You Love (or what is at least 'tolerable')

Doing what you enjoy seems like an obvious suggestion. But we rarely consider the things we love to do when we start our transformation journey. I would argue that many of us believe that if the process of transformation is not painful, then it must not be effective. I disagree. We are more concerned about doing what seemed to work for our neighbour than thinking about what we need as individuals. Perhaps we look for the magic diet and exercise combination that has been supported by some obscure research statistics or worse, endorsed by a celebrity fitness guru. We lose touch with our instincts because we aren't confident in our intuitions. We have failed so many times in the past, and that pain leaves us open to falling into the trap of doing what other people think we need to do to be healthy. Most failures occur because we don't consider the root of our weight problems or the preparation needed to succeed in the face of our underlying issues. Because of this, most of us have lost touch with our own self. Regaining that connection is essential for the recovery of our health. Reconnecting is what I am asking you to do when I suggest doing what you love to do or at least what you can find satisfaction in rather than trying to fit yourself into some weight-loss success box.

Let's look at another an example story, and afterwards I will introduce specific actions you can take to become autotelic in your health.

The story of Janice

Janice is like most of you who are reading this book. She is getting to the age where she recognizes the effects of her lifelong accumulation of poor decision making, and she desperately wants to be healthy and fit. She has wanted to achieve this feat for decades, but like most of us, she has failed in her previous attempts. Janice goes back and forth between periods of being inspired to change and feelings of defeat. She gets stuck in this cycle of short term inspiration for change, frustration, and acceptance of poor health over and over again. Each time Janice makes a new attempt to get healthy, she does what most of us do. She sees what method is out there that seems to be working for other people, and she copies it. She might pick up a fitness magazine while at the grocery store to see what the Hollywood elite is up to or make the critical error of buying a health book from an uninformed Hollywood celebrity aiming to capitalize on their fame. Perhaps Janice will hop on one of her social media outlets and find the latest Instagram star or youtube sensation who seems to have successfully gone through his or her transformation. In any case, Janice then begins to mimic the actions of her new fitness role model. Without any real thought, Janice picks someone to follow, and she begins to do what that person claims was their path to success.

It is also commonplace to do what friends or relatives do, which is often an equally poor decision. This time, Janice begins her transformation process by following Suzy's advice. Suzy is a social media fitness enthusiast whose constant flaunting of her physical assets gives the impression of health and fitness expertise. Janice eats what Suzy eats, and she does the exercises Suzy does. Everything is going well for the first few weeks, and Janice is down a few pounds. "Success," Janice thinks. But after the initial stages, Janice's mimicking of Suzy's daily actions becomes difficult. Janice is eating spinach and kale four times per day, but she *hates* intense tasting greens. Eating raw greens (which is critical for success in Suzy's opinion) makes Janice's stomach sore. Regardless of the pain and suffering, if it is what Suzy does, Janice believes she must do it too. The 15 miles Janice runs each week as per Suzy's plan is making her knees hurt so badly that she is taking anti-inflammatories just to keep up with Suzy's running schedule. Even with taking the expensive collagen supplement that Suzy has been pushing on her Instagram account, Janice is suffering from unbearable knee pain after her runs. After a month of debilitatingly sore knees and extreme gut dysfunction, Janice quits Suzy's fitness success guide and goes back to accepting her unhealthy lifestyle. The cycle begins again. Janice's health will suffer until it becomes too much to bear, and then she will try another fitness strategy that may work for someone else, but not for her.

Do you see the problem here? Doing what appears to

have worked for another person is rarely going to produce the same result in you. Even if you assume the method a fitness guru uses to look like the airbrushed version of themselves you see on the internet is what they is selling you, you are not them. If you force yourself to be like another person to take control of your health, you will most likely fail, for myriad reasons. The people we follow and mimic in an effort to succeed are rarely experts and almost always uninformed. Even if the person you follow is sincere, you likely don't have the same goals, genetics, or resources as that person. You are not helping yourself by trying to do the things they do to get in shape. My personal pre-internet equivalent of this occurred when I was a 14-year-old, skinny, insecure boy. I'd buy every bodybuilding magazine I could afford and follow the plans used by some of the world's great bodybuilders. I'd take the creatine and protein snacks they'd suggest and do every exercise in the magazine, right down to the sets and reps, in the hopes that I could look like the guy on the cover. That didn't happen. At the time, I didn't realize that the "supplementation" routine of these role models consisted of thousands of dollars a month of steroids and other potent anabolic drugs. They didn't get where they were solely from exercise and creatine. That's just the story they wanted told me, and I bought it hook, line, and sinker. I was not those men. I did not have their genes, I did not have their history, and I did not take their drugs, yet I expected to look like them by following their superficial workout plans.

Don't be fooled by the success stories that online gurus post of their clients. If you have a hundred to a thousand people following a weight loss "method," all it takes is 5% of those people to see some success to create social proof. It doesn't take a lot of progress to pretend to have a successful method. But you should not buy into exceptions.

There are always going to be a few people who succeed in doing what someone else has done, but this is the tiny minority. The minority will be so happy with their success that they will be obnoxiously loud in spreading the word about what they followed. This is how things like the Paleo Diet, plant-based diets, the Ketogenic Diet, and now the carnivore diet, explode in popularity. All diets will work for a certain percentage of the population, but it can seem as though it is working for everyone who tries it. Don't get me wrong; I am not suggesting that these diets can't be helpful or don't have value. I would say that each has a lot to offer the average person, but ideological diets are rigid and dogmatic. Groups who push them do not account for the fact that as much as human beings are alike, we are also different. If we don't account for individuality, we decrease our chances of success.

So lesson #1 in this section is not to do what someone else did and assume that you will achieve the same results. You need to be aware of this because people who *have* succeeded while following a particular weight-loss trend will be preachy. The connection between most diets and individual achievements they produce is a correlation, not a causation. In other words, the weight-loss method used by a few successful people is more of a coincidence than it is the core reason for their success.

When you implement diet and exercise approaches, you must understand how they are going to work for you, individually, and you can't try to fit yourself into another person's box. Much like forcing a square peg into a round hole, it just isn't going to work out no matter how hard you push it.

Success is not about the details of the program structure. Success in dietary approaches is simply a matter of timing. When someone is in a place where they are ready to change, and all of the pieces are in place, they will succeed with almost any dietary structure. Someone who follows the principles in this book and has a scaffolding for success can follow Paleo, vegan, high carb, low carb, high protein, or high-fat approaches. Once you are disciplined and self-aware, it all comes down to individualization and personal preference. When you are in a place where success is inevitable, the dietary structure you choose to follow is more about personal philosophy than it is about dietary technicalities. This is the point I was making when saying that stories of accomplishment that are attached to weight loss methods are nothing more than a coincidence. That goes for my clients as well. Our success stories are a result of psychological shifts made in the mindset of our members. The fact that our accomplished clients are following our particular diet and exercise guidance at the time of their success is the least important factor. Develop the proper success mindset and the details of your diet and exercise program will not matter, as long as you eat whole foods, control your intake, and move your body.

Don't let scientism sway you from your intuition

sci·en·tism
/ˈsīənˌtizəm/

noun
1. **thought or expression regarded as characteristic of scientists.**
   - ○ **excessive belief in the power of scientific knowledge and techniques.**

Throughout the book, I have sprinkled in my opinion regarding unprofessional and uneducated fitness gurus: those who make ridiculous, glorified claims about the effectiveness of their weight loss schemes. At the opposite end of the spectrum, we have the scientism crowd, and worse, stupid people who believe they understand science. Scientism suggests that what happens in a Petri dish can be extrapolated to something useful in practice. I find "Scientism" to be interchangeable with the term "evidence-based." In both cases, researchers or fitness professionals believe that reductionistic statistics are going to lead to the best health outcomes in the real world, and that any strategy that wasn't examined under a microscope can't have value. I am not suggesting that science, research, and testing are not crucial for progress - they are - but science can prevent progress as well. When suggestions derived from a microscope are generalized to lifestyle advice, there will be a disconnect.

When scientism prevents progress

Most scientists and researchers in the world of health and fitness conduct studies to gain evidence. Evidence then results in further research to test the strength of the predicted outcome. This process is repeated until a conclusion can be drawn. Most researchers do not conduct these experiments to make definitive and rigid claims about their findings. However some are out to make headlines. The average person will read these, and believe them to be literal and applicable to their life. Here are some examples of things we used to think that caused human beings great harm.

- Bloodletting is a valid medical intervention for a

variety of ailments

- Smoking is safe- even for pregnant women

- Refined sugar is part of a healthy diet

- Consuming fat (like butter) will result in heart disease

- Eggs are as damaging as cigarettes to human health

The list goes on. You may have noticed that some researchers still push some of the examples above. Publishing lousy science and shocking headlines usually stems from a desire to get attention for research.

When fitness people misrepresent good science

The rubber meets the road when inconclusive or weak studies get into the hands of casual fitness people. Let's say I have forty clients that I am working with, and I have all of those clients focus on getting 8 hours of sleep per night. This seems like a reasonable lifestyle goal to support their weight loss efforts. As nightly sleep increases, the vast majority of my clients lose a significant amount of weight. They also find it easier to make healthy decisions on a day-to-day basis because improved sleep results in better cognitive resilience. I can conclude that focusing on sleep quality achieves better results, even if these results in my clients are entirely anecdotal. I didn't have them sleep in a lab or put them in a calorimeter or have a comparison group. I simply made a suggestion and saw a typical positive result.

Imagine that the following week, a new study comes out with a headline that reads, "Increased sleep time results in a higher incidence of stroke." That is an actual headline from research that has been circulating in the popular media. Every casual personal trainer and Instagram fitness model begins sharing the study with their network telling people, "Sleep less. Your life depends on it! See, I have a study that says so!" Workaholics and hyper-performers rejoice at the news, and now my clients are questioning whether sleeping eight hours or more per night is going to kill them. Even though they lost weight, felt great, and showed improved self-control with longer sleep duration, they now call it all into question because of a headline taken too far. Nobody bothered asking why the group studied was sleeping so long in the first place. Why were people having trouble getting out of bed? Was the group so low in energy that they required ten hours of sleep per night? Were many of them depressed? What causes a person to spend excessive hours in bed? A rational person would wonder if the time in bed was a symptom of an underlying issue that could be the actual mechanism for an increased risk of stroke. But that isn't how this stuff works. In popular science media, you find a casual association, and then you cherry-pick the conclusion that will get you the most clicks. The most popular current example of this associative issue is with red meat.

Claim: Red Meat increases the risk of disease.

Logic: In populations where people ate more red meat, processed meat, and fast food, and drank more, smoked more, and exercised less, we concluded that increased disease risk must be due to red meat consumption — not all of those other factors.

Prior to the red meat deomonization, fat intake was named as the most significant risk factor for heart disease in the era of Ancel Keys. Sugar companies were paying major journals for the privelage of handpicking studies which took the heat off of 'big sugar' and directed it to 'big fat'. Now, in the updated dietary guidelines, the limitation on fat intake has been silently removed, and a limit on sugar intake was added. This just goes to show how confused scientists are about nutrition.

What about the science of weight loss supplements?

If you want to see the most long-standing example of how science is abused in fitness, look no further than the claims made by supplement manufacturers. I know most scientists would not consider these companies to be making use of very much science. Still, the average person might struggle to distinguish between what someone in a lab coat says on a supplement ad and what someone in a lab coat says inside a laboratory. Claims like, "This protein powder is shown to increase protein synthesis by 83%", or "Our patented combination of natural herbs is shown to increase fat burning by 300%" are standard in supplement advertisements. Look no further than multi-level marketing giant, Isagenix, and their cleansing claim, "This cleansing and fat burning 'starter pack' is ideal for individuals who want to lose weight using a **long-term**, flexible program. The system is a groundbreaking path to healthy weight loss and is also designed to help support the body's natural detoxification systems." The product description was taken directly from the company website. Isagenix has the nerve to use the phrases "long-term" and "healthy" to describe a thirty-day, ultra low-calorie meal replacement product. All you need to do is eat significantly fewer meals, consume far fewer calories, and spend over $400 on their "scientifically backed" shake system. Don't worry, though. They used a study to back up their claims. The study was funded by Isagenix, where the difference in result between the Isagenix group and the control group was negligible. This is a great example of abusing "science" to prey on desperate weight loss seekers.

Valid research that doesn't account for real life

What about legitimate research that suggests sprinting is more effective than walking, squats are more effective than push-ups, and free weights are more effective than machines when considering exercise selection for weight loss? Are these the details that make the difference in our fitness? Have we just been missing the magic supplement or performing ineffective exercises for fat burning and muscle building all this time? Science rarely accounts for practicality, and what happens in a beaker is unlikely to happen in your body. Let's explore this further with a story about Jack.

Jack wants to get "jacked"

Jack is in his mid-twenties and is looking to become fit. He is not particularly athletic, but he has some experience in the gym. Jack works out three days a week and does whatever he feels like on each particular day. He supports his gym activities with some jogging a few days a week and casual walks when he has the time. He is active, and he enjoys the time he spends exercising both inside and outside the gym.

It has been a few months of a steady routine, and Jack is feeling pretty good. He's lost a few pounds of fat and can see some new muscles that weren't there before. He is beginning to feel inspired to take his fitness to the next level. Jack starts to read about how to make his workouts more effective for fat loss and muscle gain. After many hours of research, Jack begins to question everything he has been doing on his transformation journey. It turns out that running isn't that great for you. According to the latest article, running burns away muscle and damages your knees. Walking doesn't burn a lot of calories and is seemingly a waste of time, according to a famous online guru. And according to a friend's performance journal article, the isolated machine exercises Jack has been doing don't produce nearly the same amount of new muscle fibres as compound movements. Jack has been doing everything incorrectly!

After hours of internet investigation, Jack changes everything he has been doing. He doesn't jog anymore. That is a one-way ticket to skinny, not muscular arms and legs. Now he only performs sprint intervals on the treadmill at a precise incline that activates the "teardrop" muscle in his quadriceps better. He has traded his walking lunges and dumbbell presses for back squats and deadlifts. His walks are nothing more than a waste of time, so why would he waste a few hours each week on this low-intensity style of exercise? Instead of his weekly walks, Jack decides to follow an at-home 20-minute fat-burning circuit in his basement that is inspired by the most recent evidence of energy systems training. Jack is a new man. An evidence obsessed man.

A few months go by, and Jack looks excellent. He has put on a few pounds of muscle, and people are beginning to take notice. It seems as though his plan to follow the path of the most effective exercise methods is working for him. Success! But not so fast. While Jack is looking better than he did a month ago, he feels terrible, both physically and mentally. His lower back is getting sore and dysfunctional from all the squatting and deadlifting that he has been doing. He needs to take a few weeks to recover enough to get another workout in. Now that Jack doesn't jog, he spends most of his cardio time in the stuffy gym, and he misses getting out into the woods and clearing his head with his trail runs.

Walking was once something that allowed Jack to relax and reconnect with himself after a long, stressful day. Still, he doesn't have time for casual walking anymore since he implemented the effective fat-burning basement workouts. Jack is looking better, but he is deteriorating physically and mentally deteriorating. He gets so psychologically burnt out and physically beat up by trying to keep up with the "effective approach" to fitness that he finally has to take three months off from the gym. He loses all the muscle he built, his back is a mess, and Jack is worse off than he was before he started casually exercising. If Jack had stuck to doing what he enjoyed from the start, imagine where it would have taken him. A year from now or even five years from now, he would surely be in excellent health. Instead, Jack may never step foot in the gym again because he felt pressured to do what the magazines, gurus, and Instagram stars told him to do.

I am by no means trying to offend fitness experts. I am aware that deadlifting and squatting do not inherently cause back problems. I am using these examples to make an important point: when we give up the activities we love doing for what are touted to be more effective methods of diet or exercise, we lose ourselves. We are swayed by the evidence-based and scientism crowds.

I see this all the time in the fitness industry from both legitimate practitioners and casual fitness personalities. How many times have you heard conversations like this:

Person 1: "I run five days a week."

Professional: "Oh, that's your problem. Steady-state cardio has a high demand and gives little return. It is highly catabolic and will eat away at your muscle."

Or

Person 1: "I've started eating a lot more fruits, vegetables, and whole grains."

Paleo nutritionist: "Oh, that's your problem. You're probably spiking your insulin with all of those carbohydrates, especially the fruit, and the insulin response is preventing you from burning fat."

These statements are scientifically accurate in some cases, but unhelpful when it comes to real-life applications of the science. An appropriate response would be, "Hey, that's awesome that you are running five days per week and adding in whole foods to your diet, keep it up!"

If you sacrifice the healthy actions that bring joy to your life for things deemed "more effective" by someone who is not you and does not know anything about you, you will eventually suffer. If not now, next month. If not next month, next year. What is "most effective" will never get you as far as what you can fit into your life in the most balanced way. This is because sustainability wins the game, and what you love to do is what you will continue for the most extended period.

Why Sustainability Matters

Since we are on the topic of 'balance' and what fits into your life, we should cover the importance of perpetual sustainability. Perpetual sustainability is the idea that any action you can perform and maintain for the rest of your life is ideal. One you cannot stick to is worthless, at least when it comes to maintaining a healthy lifestyle. We talked about this casually in a few sections of this chapter. This concept is as simple as it is accurate. Lack of sustainability is why I often speak out against "detoxes," "resets," and methods that force unnatural and unsustainable weight loss results in a concentrated period, usually by masking forms of substantial caloric restriction as "detoxification." It's relatively easy to lose a significant amount of weight in a short period with unsustainable food restriction. Call it a "cleanse" or a "reset," but we all know these products are being sold as weight loss products. If only it were as simple as having a giant bowel movement or shedding mass toxins to change your body. Maybe you try one of these cleanses, and you lose seven pounds in a week. That sounds like something to get excited about, but you'd better be prepared to see the return of that seven pounds in about a week because the weight loss is an illusion. This is where they get you. What most people don't know is that when calories are greatly restricted or replaced with shakes and supplements, the vast majority of the weight that is lost is in the form of water, glycogen, muscle, and digestive weight. It isn't fat you are losing. Your only solution to this issue of detox relapse is to buy another detox supplement. You do a 14-30 day cleanse, you lose some weight. The cleanse ends, you gain the weight back, and so, you buy another cleanse. You repeat the cycle, never getting anywhere except into a hyper yo-yo dieting cycle that never establishes any long term results. Welcome to the product-based weight loss solution market!

When I do speaking engagements, I often ask the question, "By a show of hands, how many of you have tried a dietary approach that worked for you?" At least half of the room will put their hands up. Then I follow up with this statement, "Keep in mind that when I say 'worked for you,' I mean you have kept the peak of your results up until today." At this point, zero hands remain in the air. **Any action that you cannot maintain for the rest of your life will not produce long-term results. Results come from daily operations, not from isolated, temporary, unsustainable activities**. Healthy actions are not "scalable"; you must perform them regularly to maintain your success. Believing otherwise is like suggesting that you can give up brushing your teeth by getting fluoride treatment from your dentist once a year. Sure, the fluoride treatment *might* be helpful, but the daily brushing and flossing of your teeth are what keep up dental hygiene. The rest of your body operates the same way. In all areas of your life, benefits that you gain will only be sustained by continuing the daily rituals that got you there in the first place.

Anyone can grind it out for 30 days

This brings us to an essential point that it is the basis for so many fallacies in the health and fitness world. It is the source of so many "snapshot" success stories that companies use to promote the effectiveness of a product or method. Even though the subjects of most success stories have not maintained the result that is being promoted in the ad or social account, you certainly don't know that. Fleeting "social proof" is one of the reasons why resets, detoxes, cleanses, and "30-day challenges" are so appealing to people. You see a product, you see a person like you, and you witness that person's extreme success. This pushes you to try the product or program. But here's the catch: anyone can do anything for 30 days, regardless of how torturous the process might be. And within that 30 days, you can see some dramatic results if you are only consuming 750 calories of liquid nutrition per day and exercising your butt off. But those results seldom remain in the long term. Once the picture is snapped, and a person's extreme transformation is documented, what happens to that person's body afterward is no longer relevant. You only see the result of short term suffering. You don't witness the result of the long-term relapse.

As I mentioned at the beginning of the chapter, **there is unlimited evidence showing that people can tolerate an extreme amount of discomfort, as long as they know the timeline of the suffering.** This is especially true when the timeline is short. When the schedule is uncertain (or certainly long), we don't do so well. The ability to suffer when the duration of the suffering is understood is a well-studied concept in psychology. In animals, stress hormones and agitation go through the roof when electrical shocks or feeding schedules are random. When the pattern (of both positive and negative stimuli) are routine, the suffering of the animal is much less. In humans, studies like these have been performed in jail-like scenarios. When test subjects are confined and isolated for a pre-determined period, stress levels are controlled. When the subject has no idea what the duration of the isolation will be, stress levels are very high.

This mindset explains why so many of us determined to torture ourselves to achieve the results we want. We much prefer restriction for four to twelve weeks to making more reasonable changes for an undetermined period. When a certain amount of weight loss is promised to us in a concentrated timeline, we can do almost anything. Our psychological biases are being exploited. This is a widespread and effective industry tactic.

What is the remedy to this psychological heuristic? This is where the "less is more" approach comes in. If you want to succeed, you need to understand that partaking in extreme, torturous processes in the hopes of getting quick results is not realistic. You would be much better off by focusing on small actions that you can take each day that will, over time, accumulate and bring you long term results. Sometimes it is better to walk than it is to run by integrating small, enjoyable changes into your life. See what small actions can do for you a year from now. As soon as someone comes to me and says, "I need to lose 'X' amount of weight by 'Y' date, and I am considering following 'Z' approach to do it," I know this person is going to fail. That person is going to be having the same conversation with someone like me at this time next year because nothing will have changed. Unfortunately, humans are present biased, so this is an uphill battle for all of us. Being "present biased" means we give up positive long-term results in exchange for short term gambles or immediate gratification. When you eat ten cookies even though cookie consumption is not helping your 6-month weight loss goal, you are acting on your present bias. When you give up on small, practical, routine exercise and dietary interventions for a lemon and cayenne pepper water cleanse, you are acting on a version of this bias as well. When a client of mine becomes frustrated and is on the verge of giving up, I suggest to her, "Think about yourself a year from now looking back at this moment. Next year you can reflect and say 'I shouldn't have quit. I can only imagine where I would be right now if I had kept up my small, daily healthy habits' or you can look back and say, 'I'm so glad I kept this up. I'm down 40 pounds, and I couldn't be happier'." I attempt to frame her mind to allow her to get past her present bias. In challenging moments, we must overcome our yearning for immediate results. If three years ago, you had decided to commit to small actions each day regardless of the direct outcome, you would be an entirely different version of yourself today. It reminds me of a thought experiment I use in my own life when I struggle to make positive decisions for my future self.

Many of us feel like we are too old to commit to anything that won't give us results in a short-term period. But tomorrow, next year, and the next decade are still going to come. So, which version of yourself would you like to be at that time? For instance, let's say you're 48 years old. If I told you it would take five years for you to reach your goal, you would be discouraged. You wouldn't see the value in changing your lifestyle, and you wouldn't even start trying. But in five years you're still going to be 53 years old, and you're still going to be either slim and healthy, or sick and overweight. So which version of yourself do you want to be in five years? One version will leave you feeling proud, confident, and happy. The other version will leave you sad, regretful, and afraid. If you practiced this thinking for the last five years, today you would be so successful that you would not even be reading this book. So who are you going to be five years *after* reading this book? That all depends on which mindset you choose.

If there is anything I want you to take away from this chapter, it is the encouragement to do what you love instead of doing what someone convinces you is effective-especially if what is "effective" pulls you away from what you love to do. I want you to do the small, seemingly insignificant daily actions you value instead of getting sucked into the quick-fix products and methods that promise results that never actually stick in the long-term. You must overcome your present bias and the desire to see health as something that you need to achieve in a rapid time frame. It is impossible to achieve sustainable health outcomes in the short term, so you might as well look at the long run and fill your days with small, healthy actions that bring joy and satisfaction to your life. That is what being autotelic is really about. You find the steps that contribute to your goals as well as your overall wellbeing. As you build on these habits, over time, you become successful without even realizing it. If you implement the daily, healthy actions that you would be happy to pursue, even if they never lead to a single pound lost on the scale, that is when the needle begins to move. Much like Mr.Gates and Ms.Adele would be fiddling with computers and belting out ballads even if it never earned either of them a penny, you must learn to take care of your body through ways that bring you joy, not just results. Being results-centric leads to disappointment and self-sabotage. Being action-centric and rewarding yourself for being kind to your body and mind will lead to results and fulfillment.

In an industry of confusion and information overload it's easy to second guess ourselves. When wondering what is better for you, Yoga or CrossFit, the answer should not be outsourced to another person's opinion. It should be internal. The question should be, "What do I enjoy more, Yoga, or CrossFit"? If the answer is "yoga," yoga is more effective. If the answer is "CrossFit," CrossFit is more effective. If all you like to do is walk, then walk. Walk every day. You need to use this system of internal questioning for every health decision you make.

If you fill your days with healthy choices that you would continue making regardless of the result, you will attain a result that you would never have otherwise accomplished.

Key Takeaways

- *Actions must be self-rewarding (autotelic) if you are going to keep them up*
- *Efforts should be your measurement of success, not the scale*
- *Do things you enjoy first (or which you can best tolerate)*
- *The degree of change is less important than repetition. The small things you do every day will take you further than large efforts that you struggle to do consistently*

Everyone needs to have a goal, but when the goal is specific, arbitrary, and with a timeline, we suffer. It is much better to focus on lead measures. Lead measures are the things you need to do to hit the superficial goal. Lead measures are also actions that should be most rewarding and celebrated. Making more of your own meals, exercising daily, and reducing snacking are the kinds of lead measures that you should undertake. It would help if you also spent more time doing healthy stuff that you enjoy rather than things someone told you would give you results, but you hate doing. Success comes from taking small, repeatable actions, not from taking big giant leaps toward your goal.

CHAPTER 7- SUCCESS LEVERS OF LIFESTYLE

"With adequate sleep, half of the weight the dieters lost was from fat, not muscle, and furthermore, those on a sleep-deprived diet experienced 55% less fat loss. The sleep-deprived group also felt significantly hungrier, had less satisfaction after meals, and lacked enough energy to exercise. There are a few biological mechanisms that explain why not sleeping enough can make you fat or disrupt your diet. For example, within just four days of sleep deprivation, your body's ability to properly respond to insulin signals begins to diminish (University of Chicago researchers found a 30% drop insulin sensitivity caused by lack of sleep). When you're not responsive to insulin, fat cells are far less able to release fatty acids and lipids to produce energy, blood glucose remains higher, and any extra fats and sugars circulating in your blood cause you to pump out even more insulin. Eventually, all this excess insulin causes you to begin storing fat in all the wrong places, including tissues like your liver, leading to problems such as fatty liver and diabetes."-

Summary from the annals of internal medicine

At the beginning of this book, I emphasized that being diet- and exercise- focused without establishing your underlying psychological motivations for unhealthy behaviour is a losing game. If you attempt to make diet and exercise changes without first setting the proper groundwork, you will never stick to your diet and exercise efforts in the long-term. Success becomes impossible rather than inevitable. You should now have the tools necessary to begin working on your psychological blind spots, but there is still much you can do outside of diet and exercise to maximize your chances of success. I am talking about managing your lifestyle.

So what is "lifestyle?" If you think about all of the factors outside diet and exercise that can contribute to a healthier body, most of them fall into the "lifestyle" bucket. How well we sleep, how we manage stress, and the activities we pursue and avoid in our free time are our "lifestyle." Don't worry if you have never made the connection between lifestyle factors and your body before, or if you aren't aware of how sleep quality and stress levels can determine your body fat percentage. Each of these lifestyle factors will be well defined and explained as we move through this chapter.

It is typical to obsess over your diet and exercise techniques without considering the impact that lifestyle management has on your waistline. I can tell you that without a full lifestyle overhaul, you won't get the results from your diet and exercise efforts that you otherwise could have. Perhaps it is more accurate to say that your road to success will be more difficult and have a lesser chance of long-term success without lifestyle changes. Creating a beneficial lifestyle will support your ability to break down the main barriers that were the focus of the first section of this book because when your lifestyle is advantageous, life change is just easier to manage. Life is more enjoyable. When you manage stress well, improve sleep quality, and adopt an active lifestyle, your health quickly improves.

Most of us know that we should be getting more sleep, stressing less, and moving more. But knowing doesn't inspire us to take action, at least not the way we are inspired to take action on diet and exercise. I believe this inability to focus on lifestyle improvements stems from a few reasons. The first is that most of us don't understand the impact that high stress, poor sleep, and a lack of casual activity have on our health and waistlines. We know that it's not ideal to have broken sleep at night, but we can't directly connect lack of sleep to being overweight, so sleep interventions take a back seat to diet and exercise actions. The second reason why we don't connect with our lifestyle is that we don't know where to begin. Diet and exercise, while sometimes confusing and ineffective, are also simple concepts to understand. "If I want to change my diet, I eat these foods and avoid these foods, and if I want to improve my exercise efforts, I do these exercises this many days per week." We get it when it comes to diet and exercise, but not when it comes to lifestyle factors that can also change our body.

The goal of this chapter is for you to give lifestyle efforts the same importance as you would diet and exercise. I want you to understand exactly how these areas can make or break your success, and what you can do right now to maximize your results in these areas. Working on sleep, stress management, and active rest, along with what you know about diet and exercise, will collectively increase your chances of success. That makes this section of the book one of the most crucial.

The Effects of Poor Sleep Quality

Before we begin talking about how poor sleeping patterns can derail our progress, we should talk about how most of us sleep. It's hard to believe, but you may not even know that you have a sleep problem. Worse, you might think your sleep issues are normal or even admirable. Below are the three main sleep problems I regularly see in my clients.

We stay up too late: Most of us are in the habit of staying up too late, and for no good reason. Believe it or not, this is often due to a lack of life satisfaction and purpose. When we don't feel we have accomplished very much in our day, we tend to extend our waking hours. We do this so we can feel we've gotten more out of our day. We delay our bedtime because to go to bed ends the day, which, if it has been dull and uneventful, can leave us searching for a different form of satisfaction. It's ok to feel like you need more from your day. The negative feelings we get from being unproductive are likely evolutionary mechanisms to keep us contributing to the tribe. But in this scenario, we don't finish our day with anything of value. We fill the evening with unhealthy stimulation that keeps us up at all hours of the night.

When you have a job that doesn't bring you a sense of purpose, and you lack hobbies outside work that can be fulfilling, you tend to avoid sleeping. To sleep is to end your day without a much-needed feeling of accomplishment. And if you don't have a sense of accomplishment, you will seek stimulation through food and technological distraction.

Do you know when you have had the perfect day, such as when you're visiting a new city, and you pack your entire day with exploring, walking, seeing sites, and experiencing new things? Under these circumstances, you can easily go to bed at 8:30 PM without thinking twice. But when you're at home and it's been a long day at work, and you haven't accomplished much of anything, you struggle to go to bed at a reasonable hour. You need one more show, one more youtube video, one more snack, or one more hour of cruising social media. This is a simple example of the factors and mindset that allow us to go to sleep at a reasonable hour, as well as those that make it impossible to go to bed nice and early.

We stress at night: The second reason we stay up too late is that we spend the evening thinking about all of life's worries. When our daytime tasks do not occupy our brains, we are left with nothing but the sound of our minds, and the noise can be challenging to listen to sometimes. This is why worry comes in the evening. When we occupy our minds with the stimulation of daily tasks (like work, school, being at home with the kids, etc.), our brain doesn't have room for worry. When it is the end of the day, however, and our mind is idle, it is easy to seek unhealthy stimulation. This is what I call the downtime dilemma. A vacant, unproductive mind is the enemy of a reasonable bedtime and good habits.

We have an overall lack of sleep: An early bedtime alone might not immediately qualify you for getting enough sleep. Even if you get to bed by 10 PM, you may still not be sleeping long enough. For this reason, I have separated the two issues into bedtime and sleep duration. Most people require a minimum of seven hours of sleep, but that can go as high as ten hours. Most of us need something in between, and I believe the magic number is somewhere between eight and nine hours. That means hours asleep, not just hours in your bed. Statistically, most of us are sleeping between 5-6 hours per night, which is not enough. Whether you go to bed too late, wake up too early, or "burn the candle at both ends" because you feel that is what works for your life, you are suffering. Every night that you do not get enough sleep to recover and grow prevents your body from thriving the next day.

We have broken sleep patterns: Then there are those of us who fall asleep as soon as our heads hit the pillow but then spend most of the night waking and dozing off and then waking again. We might be in bed for 10 hours, but we only end up sleeping for half of that time. "Sleep Maintenance Insomnia" is common in people with unresolved personal issues and daily concerns, as well as those who struggle with metabolic and hormonal imbalances. Sometimes the inability to stay asleep is due to something as simple as a vitamin and mineral deficiency (like calcium or magnesium) that prevents the muscle tissues in our body from properly relaxing at night. If we only measure the time between when we go to bed and when we wake up, we might think we are getting adequate sleep. But if we measure the amount of time we are actually sleeping, we might find we are well short of our fundamental sleep and regeneration needs.

There may be other factors playing a role in your overall lack of sleep quality. Still, the factors I have mentioned thus far are the main ones I see in clients. These are the issues most likely affecting you. They are also the most straightforward issues to correct, so that is where we will focus.

So what is the impact of poor sleep quality that comes via the factors we have mentioned so far? The direct physiological effects might surprise you.

What low sleep quality is doing to your biology

The effects of Leptin and Ghrelin: Leptin and ghrelin seem to be key in regulating appetite, which consequently influences the amount of body fat we store (or burn). Both leptin and ghrelin are peripheral in the mechanism but central in our brain. We secrete them throughout various parts of the body, but the main effects happen in our brains. Leptin is secreted primarily in fat cells, as well as the stomach, heart, and skeletal muscle, and leptin plays a crucial role in decreasing our hunger signals. Ghrelin is secreted primarily in the lining of the stomach and, in turn, increases hunger. Leptin and ghrelin go back and forth throughout the day, telling us when it is time to eat and stop eating. The pair also control how intense our hunger and cravings might be. Both hormones respond to how much we eat. Leptin usually correlates to fat mass in the sense that the more body fat you have, the more leptin you produce, and the less hungry you should be.

Leptin in sleep: When we aren't getting enough quality sleep, we have a reduction in the activity of the hormone leptin. Since leptin is responsible for the signalling of satiety, this is a meaningful interaction. Leptin tells your brain that you don't need to eat, and your body fat stores are adequate. It is also partially responsible for fat loss via the same signalling. So if you are sleeping poorly and your leptin signalling is affected, you are more likely to overeat, and thus, gain weight.

Ghrelin in sleep: When you get a rumbling in your stomach and your desire to eat increases, that is coming from the hormone, ghrelin. When you don't get enough sleep, your ghrelin increases, which increases your desire to eat more. There's a good chance you've noticed that the less you are sleeping, and the more exhausted you are, the more likely you are to turn to food. Leptin and ghrelin both have a role in that process.

Lowered Glucose Tolerance: Lack of sleep also leads to reduced glucose tolerance. When sugars (carbohydrates) break down into glucose, that glucose enters the bloodstream but has a difficult time getting shuttled into the tissues where it is supposed to end up. The process causes a rise in our insulin levels through a common issue named insulin resistance. A healthy, well-slept individual will use a small amount of insulin to shuttle glucose (sugar) out of the bloodstream and into places like muscle tissue, the liver, and sometimes fat storage. When glucose tolerance is low, and thus insulin resistance is high, you produce far more insulin to do the same job that a small amount of insulin would do in a healthier individual. Chronically elevated insulin levels can be responsible for a lot of nasty stuff. For the sake of your weight loss interests, let's just say that when insulin is in circulation, fat burning capability is turned off, so too much insulin hinders your ability to use stored fat for energy. This is known as the insulin switch. When insulin is on, fat burning is off. When insulin is off, fat-burning capabilities are back on. In a healthy person, insulin secretion is beneficial for performance, muscle growth, recovery, and not dying from glucose toxicity. But in an unhealthy individual who is short on sleep, the overproduction of insulin becomes maladaptive and often harmful.

Many more negative effects come from being deprived of sleep. Still, the three direct physiological effects I listed above are the ones that would likely be most concerning to you with your goal of a slimmer waist and lower body fat composition. There are also many effects of poor sleep that contribute indirectly to adverse health outcomes and a larger waistline, and we will cover those in a little while. For now, we are going to take a more in-depth look at the direct effects of stress. After we have completed the stress section, I will conclude the chapter with the indirect effects of both sleep and stress on the body.

The Effects of Poor Stress Management

At this point, you should be well aware of how in modern times, incredible amounts of stress are hurting our health. Throughout the book, we have discussed how stress leads to the drive to cope and self-medicate and how this leads to our most unhealthy and self-harming behaviours. But we haven't discussed how stress affects us on a biological level. That is what we will do in this section. First, let's recall how stress accumulates in our lives with an example of what a typical day is like for many people.

You begin your day by waking up a little late, perhaps after a few snooze button pushes because of the terrible sleep you had the night before. You had a late night of mindless T.V. watching to distract your brain from the perils of the day, and now you are paying for it with dark bags under your eyes and a lazy haze. The fast jump to your alarm clock is already giving you a rush of cortisol. You are pressed for time and stressing about being late for work, and this is only five minutes into your day. You cram a bagel into your mouth as you run out the door and hope that the roads aren't congested while you begin your commute to the office. Along your drive, you encounter inconsiderate commuters who seem like their only purpose is to prevent you from getting to work on time. Since they are stressed and rushed in their own lives, they feel compelled to cut you off and perform a variety of aggressive maneuvers. You get to work only to find out that the proposal you worked on for six months was rejected, and your nemesis, "Lazy Rhonda" down the hall, received an undeserved promotion. You can't understand how someone so incompetent could create a better marketing plan than you. You spend the rest of the long day at work sitting at a desk and staring at a computer with few breaks before making your way back home through rush hour traffic and suffering the same mental anguish you did during the morning drive. By the time you get home, you are drained and defeated. You can do nothing more than sit on the couch and contemplate your life. Your finances are poor, your friendships are dying, and you've been alone for a year with no real romantic prospects on the horizon. Who even has the energy to date the days?

Stress? That is an understatement.

Feel free to replace this grim scenario with that of the stay-at-home parent covered in spit up, chasing around a toddler who pulls every book off of the shelf and every pan out of the cupboard. You scurry behind him, trying to keep your disastrous house clean enough to prevent you from spiralling into a deep depression. Or consider the student who is feeling so much financial, parental, and academic pressure to succeed that she needs to speak to a counsellor twice a week to prevent her from jumping off a rooftop. It sounds very "doom and gloom," but this is the reality of modern life for many people. Stress is everywhere, and we don't tend to manage it well. We are not designed with the necessary equipment to deal with modern stress. When you understand the biological impacts of this accumulated stress, you realize how critical it is that you exercise stress management as much as you move your body. Chances are, however, that you are not managing stress well or even focusing on stress management because you don't recognize the impact. So what are the effects of stress?

Stress and rising Cortisol: When we face stress, we increase our production of cortisol. Cortisol is a hormone which gets us ready for danger. If someone was chasing you with a knife or if a bear was on your tail, you'd want your cortisol to spike ASAP to aid in your fight or flight mechanism. But in today's life, when we face stress, it is rarely due to physical danger and almost always due to psychological factors that are non-threatening but make us feel as if we are in danger. Public speaking, having a verbal disagreement, or seeing an almost empty bank account can all start this process. Chronically elevated levels of cortisol are connected to many diseases and are also tightly correlated to other hormonal expressions (like insulin, for instance) that can result in increased body fat.

Increased blood sugar and insulin production: When we are stressed, cortisol participates in the release of sugar into the bloodstream. This elevation in blood glucose provides us with energy to fight or flee in the face of acute danger. But when we aren't fighting anything or fleeing from anyone, we end up with a needless, maladaptive increase in circulating blood sugar. As you now know, when blood sugar rises, we need to produce insulin to get that sugar out of the blood, and when insulin is circulating, our fat burning capabilities shut down. If this process happened once or twice a day for 5 minutes, it wouldn't be a big deal. However, since most of us are chronically stressed out, this process of rising blood sugar, and the resulting insulin production, become a more significant health problem.

Digestive upset and lowered immunity: Stress also has significant adverse effects on our gut health and immune function. This is mostly due to the previously mentioned hormonal cascades that come when we are stressed, and as a result, the peripheral functions of digestion and immunity suffer. When you are stressed and activating the fight or flight system, digestion shuts down. Who has time to digest an apple while being chased by a dinosaur? We need that digestive blood to escape! When we are continually diverting blood to our gut to prepare us for potential threats, our digestive system cannot adequately perform its tasks. This means we struggle to assimilate nutrients from our food and properly digest what we have eaten. The overproduction in hormones like cortisol will also eventually suppress our healthy inflammatory and immune responses, leading to dysfunction in these areas. The issue is complex, but for the purposes of this book suffice it to say that when you are more likely to be sick and tired and less likely to be recovered and rested, you are less likely to be thriving in your diet and exercise habits.

Those are the most critical direct effects of poor sleep and stress management. Hopefully, the physiological ailments discussed are enough to inspire you to take rest and stress management more seriously. But just in case they aren't, let's look at the indirect effects as well.

The Indirect Effects of Poor Sleep and Stress Management

Direct effects are reactions that happen with simple cause and effect. For example, when you face overwhelming stress or when your sleep quality is suffering, you are going to suffer automatic pschyological and phsyiological reactions. Those are the direct effects of poor lifestyle management. Then there are secondary reactions to poor lifestyle management that lead to complicated problems in a less straightforward way. Some examples of these indirect reactions are below.

Poor decision making: When you are stressed and

deprived of sleep, you have very little room for healthy decision making. This is a significant problem. For most of us, making changes to our health requires substantial behavioural change, and behavioural change takes a lot of mental strength and discipline. Lacking the mental capacity to make the right decisions, you end up eating at the drive-thru and skipping the gym. When we are happy, full of energy, and ready to take on the world, we can make the right decisions instead of the harmful, tempting ones. But when we are stressed, tired, and barely have enough energy to sit upright, decision making takes a back seat to our unhealthy autopilot.

Low energy: When you are stressed and tired, it goes without saying that your energy levels will be deficient. When energy levels are low, you are more likely to be unproductive in your downtime, which makes you more likely to succumb to cravings and late-night eating. When 3-4 hours of your night are spent lounging around and distracting yourself with technology, food is going to play a supporting role. When you are unstimulated, unproductive, or inactive, you become trapped within the cycle of your most unhealthy behaviours.

High-calorie cravings: Lastly, when you are struggling with sleep and stress, your brain is more likely to crave things like glucose, fat, and salt, and you are more likely to be comforted by high energy foods. Your brain uses up about 25% of the glucose in your body on any given day for smooth cognitive operation. When you are particularly overwhelmed with life, your brain will ask you to increase its energy supply. This results in increased cravings for sweet, salty, fatty, high energy foods. You become more likely to make poor decisions, and you lack the energy to do the stimulating activities that can keep you away from the cookie jar. Your brain also begs you for high energy foods to soothe its issues of operation.

The Sleep and Stress Cycle

I hope my examples of the effects of poor sleep and stress management are enough to convince you of their importance. I should also touch on how the relationship between sleep and stress is an intimate one that can create a negative feedback loop. When we are suffering in one area of sleep or stress management, we are more likely to suffer in the other. A perpetual cycle of worsening symptoms in both areas of sleep and stress can result, which ends up being a compounded problem for your waistline. When you have a terrible sleep, you are more susceptible to the stress you face that day. You're tired, you're irritable, and you don't have the energy required to withstand basic adversities. As your day brings you stressful moments, you become increasingly sensitive to them; each new stress worsens the situation. If you began your day tired and cranky, smaller pressures can affect you just as much as a substantial stressor would on a day when you slept well the night before. When you finally get home and have the opportunity to relax, these mounting stresses prevent you from proper decompression. The result is late nights of eating and distracting due to a mind plagued by anxiety, frustration, and anger. The accumulated stresses can even cause hormonal disruptions that break up your sleep cycles. These stress-induced late nights and broken sleep patterns lead to lower sleep quality, and lower sleep quality leads to increased sensitivity to stress the next day. When the morning comes, you are starting with a higher sensitivity to stress than you were the day before. By the end of the day, you won't be in a position to properly decompress and recover with proper sleep quality and duration. Each day you are running a race with only one leg and trying to catch up to the pack. It can be a vicious reality to deal with, and if you do not correct the pattern, diet and exercise changes will be challenging to retain.

When Good Stress Becomes Bad Stress

The last thing I want to note before moving on is how "good stress" can become "bad stress." We have come to know exercise to be "good stress." We overload the body with some sort of physical stimulus (lifting a weight, for example) that our muscle has to struggle to raise. The stress of lifting forces the body to respond by increasing the number of muscle fibres that move the weight, and in the process, these fibres are damaged. Our body adapts to that stress by increasing the size or amount of our muscle fibres when repairing the damage, and this is how we build strength and new muscle. This is known as "eustress." In a healthy individual, this is a positive process. But is this true when we are short on sleep and overstressed? While there is definitely "good stress" that we can place on the body, it is still a contributor to our overall accumulation of total stress. When our system is overwhelmed with stress, the "good stress" equals more load on the mind and body.

Good stress makes us distressed. This can make activities like intense exercise become a negative stimulus on the body. Think of your capacity to deal with stress as a bucket. The overflowing of that bucket is an adverse health outcome due to stress overload. If your bucket is ¼ full of harmful stress, you have lots of room for proper pressures that give you a positive health response without needing to worry about an overflow of total demand. But, if you have a bucket that is ¾ full of bad stress, even a few drops of good stress is eventually going to cause the bucket to overflow, at which point the good to lousy stress ratio doesn't matter. You are facing too much overall stress, and you are distressed. So the last negative effect of the poor sleep and stress management complex is that the accumulation of bad stress prevents us from benefiting from the positive pressure in our lives. It can make something as useful as exercise problematic with injury, metabolic issues, and degeneration. This is why those who try to overexercise and undereat to tackle a weight problem often suffer dramatic rebounds and even severe health consequences. Eating too little is a stress on the body. Exercising too much is a stress on the body. Add in your poorly managed life stress and your poor sleep quality, and your body will revolt or shut down.

Sleep and stress are crucial lifestyle factors that must be addressed to create long-term sustainable results in your health. Daily sleep and stress exercises should fit into your long-term weight loss plan, just like your diet and exercise interventions do. Approaching all of these health factors in combination will increase your rate of success exponentially. Now that we have looked at the complex factors in great depth, let's move on to the final lifestyle management factor: becoming a genuinely active human being.

Being a Genuinely Active Person

Many of us believe that we are active because we go to the gym 2-4 days per week. We label ourselves as "active" individuals for a handful of the 168 hours in our week we bust our butts with intense activity. I'm not trying to minimize your gym efforts, and I think it is excellent when any person commits to the gym. Intense exercise has many benefits that should not be understated or undermined. But going to the gym a few hours per week does not make you "active" any more than eating 1-2 healthy meals in a week of 20-30 meals makes you a healthy eater. If you ate fast food 20 times per week but had 5-10 home-cooked meals as well, would be a healthy eater? Not likely. We tend to remember the few times we make it to the gym while forgetting about the 40+ hours we spent sitting at a desk or on the couch, perhaps while eating. If you want to succeed in your transformation, you must begin filling your day with meaningful activity in place of your typical unproductive and sedentary habits. You don't need to be extreme about it, but there are little things you can start doing right now that will give you high returns with minimal effort. There are many activities you can do that are simple, easy, and free that will contribute just as much or more to your overall health than formal exercise alone. I will break these down.

The Power of N.E.A.T.

N.E.A.T. stands for non-exercise activity thermogenesis. The activity refers to the things you do that are not formally planned exercise. Thermogenesis is the production of heat. Examples of NEAT activities are frequently getting up from your seated position to stretch or move around, and taking the stairs instead of the escalator. Most of us disregard these forms of energy expenditure because we see them as insignificant. Still, those of us who have high daily NEAT scores will burn more calories through NEAT than through formal exercise at the gym. The effects of NEAT are significant. Movement opportunities come up often and don't require the need for rest, recovery, planning, or scheduling. This is in contrast to activities like going to the gym or taking part in formal types of exercise that require specific time dedication and periods of recovery. If you begin to be aware of these NEAT opportunities (like not fighting for the closest parking spot when you go to the grocery store), you could accumulate 300-500 extra calories expended per day. That is a significant amount of energy you're using, and most of it is from fat, so don't turn your back on these undercover exercises. NEAT can be a crucial part of your total daily health plan.

Active Rest

Active rest is a form of planned exercise that you do more for joy or recovery than you do for burning muscles and lungs. Going for a long walk, doing some light Yoga or mobility in your basement or the backyard, or even more obscure forms of light exercise like Tai Chi would all be considered types of active rest. Much like NEAT, active rest does not require a specific appointment, place, or period of recovery. You can do it anywhere, anytime, and not need to worry about how it affects your formal exercise sessions. If you're about to turn on the T.V., you could always go outside for a walk instead. This is what active rest is all about. Much like NEAT, active rest has a significant impact on your overall caloric expenditure. For instance, a 200 lb 40-year-old female can burn around 300 calories just from an hour of walking. That doesn't even take into account the psychological benefits of fresh air, nature, and time to think! It doesn't matter what you do, just as long as you aim to do some form of active rest each day, or as often as you can be inspired to do it.

Active rest and the "downtime dilemma"

The "downtime dilemma" is a situation where many of us end up undoing most of our results. A typical example of the downtime dilemma is getting home from work or school. Dinner is over, and all you want to do is sit down and relax. For most of us, this time is between 6 PM and 12 AM. During this time, we watch T.V., scroll through our smartphones, or cruise social networking on our laptop. If we're honest, most of us are doing at least two of the three at once in a very mindless way. The result is giving into unconscious cravings during this window of time. Late-night snacking, overeating, laziness, and many of our significant unhealthy behaviours are driven by the uncomfortable boredom mechanism or anxious emotions. Painful feelings arise while our mind is idling during these uninteresting activities. The hours we spend mindlessly relaxing leave our mind craving stimulation, and when looking for stimulation, our brain asks for food and other unhelpful distractions. Most of us would agree that this is the time of day where we take part in uncontrolled and unhealthy actions.

Active rest can be a great fix for this issue. Getting up off the couch can sometimes feel like more effort than it is worth, but going for a short walk, doing some light stretching or getting in our meditation and breathing exercises will get us away from our worst habits. These are techniques to save us from ourselves. Productive stimulation energizes us more than melting into the couch does. Some people feel like resting is the key to recovery, but it is active rest that gives us the highest return. Considering we use the need to "decompress and reenergize" as our excuse to watch Netflix all night long, it is helpful to understand that T.V. watching is energy-sucking while active rest is energy-creating. When we further contribute to our health, rather than hurt it with uncontrollable snacking, we feel better about ourselves, and our mood improves. This improvement in mood makes it easier to sleep at night and reduces our feelings of stress and anxiety before bedtime. You know how valuable sleep hygiene can be after reading the earlier sections of this chapter. It is all connected. Active rest isn't just a contributor to caloric expenditure. It is also an indirect contributor to snacking control, stress reduction, and improved sleep quality. Becoming a truly active person can change your health and body more than the time you spend torturing yourself in the gym.

Putting work into this area of your health plan will give you returns beyond what you would ever picture in your mind. I hope I have convinced you that a combination of all of the factors mentioned in this book is the key to your health. All the aspects of your well-being that I've covered up until this point are closely interconnected. Remember that sleep affects stress, stress affects sleep, and both affect your sensitivity and need to self-medicate. All of these factors influence your ability to make the right food decisions. You are much better off putting a little bit of effort into every area of your life than you are obsessing over any single aspect like diet or exercise. We put all of our eggs into one basket and then wonder why it always comes crashing down around us. Synergy is the key to maximal success in health, and if you approach each factor in this chapter like you would your diet and exercise efforts, you will begin to see where long-term results come from.

Key Takeaways

· *Poor sleep and high stress lead to weight gain, both directly and indirectly.*

· *Being genuinely active on a consistent basis is better than being intensely active in spurts and lazy the rest of the time.*

· *Your downtime habits must be changed if you are going to overcome your most unhealthy behaviours.*

The foods you eat and the exercises you do matter to your health. Sleep quality and stress management matter just as much, if not more than diet and activity. Sleeping well, reducing stress, and increasing casual activity have both direct and indirect effects on your waistline that matter. If you can improve these areas of your lifestyle, healthy choices become more comfortable and give higher returns.

CHAPTER 8- TRAIN THE BRAIN FOR CHANGE

"Between stimulus and response there is a space. In that space is our power to choose our response. In our response lies our growth and our freedom."
— Viktor E. Frankl

At this point in the book, it is safe to assume that you understand the value of your mindset. Your mindset can promote physiological improvements, including your ability to lose weight. In this chapter, I am going to teach you the most effective techniques to train your brain, just like you would train your body. Brain training aims to increase the strength and resilience of your mind to ensure you set yourself up for long-term success. Without an improved mindset, diet and exercise interventions will not help you. You can use the strategies discussed in this chapter to help manage stress, control cravings, and commit to going to the gym. Any actions you need to take or break to succeed will be easier to apply with these tools. The techniques in this chapter will aid in making specific improvements in areas where you have struggled in the past. Meaningful behavioural change is the key to accumulating the necessary positive choices that lead to substantial long term results, so get out your notepad!

The importance of objectification

Whether we are dealing with a stressful situation, are bogged down in an overwhelming emotion, or are mindlessly eating sweet and salty snacks, there is a trend. We are ignoring reality. We are letting the stress, emotion, and unhealthy coping take hold of our mind. Take a stressful situation, for instance. You are driving home after a long day at work, and out of nowhere, a car comes flying up behind you. The careless driver does this in an attempt to encourage you to move more quickly. You don't succumb to such intimidation tactics and maintain your speed. So the driver peels around you as quickly as she can, rolls down her window, and screams an expletive as she blows by and flies down the road. How are you most likely to react to this situation? Chances are your face will get red and hot. Your pulse will increase, and you will begin to picture a scenario in which this person skids out of control and ends up in a ditch. You may even imagine slowly driving by and casually waving at her in her moment of suffering. What about 2 hours after the incident? You continue to replay this interaction in your mind, so much so that you continue to think about this horrible human being the next day. At this point, her yelling is the least that this person has done to you. Since the incident, she has taken up real estate in your mind, and you have allowed it. The rumination is spiking your cortisol and increasing your chronic stress long after the incident ended. This is classified as letting the stress live within you.

How about a food-based example of this problem? It's Saturday night, and you decide to stay in and relax with a movie. You turn on a show and grab a few indulgences to snack on during the movie. The snacks don't last quite as long and as you anticipated, and you find yourself popping out to the pantry for a small bag of chips. Then again, for a bag of popcorn. Then some cookies. Then some crackers. It's only 45 minutes into the movie, and you are on consumption autopilot. You can't even remember how the last thing you ate tasted. Bites blend and snacks merge into a blur. The two-hour-long snacking session becomes a lucid dream that you can barely recall. The only way you piece together the amount of food you consumed is by the gnawing, sore feeling you have in your stomach. You lost all sense of presence while eating in front of the T.V. screen and mindlessly devoured every snack in your cupboard. You can barely even remember how it all started. Your craving took hold and dictated your actions. The craving was living deep within your subconscious. How else could you have allowed such excess?

These are examples of internalization, the opposite of objectification. Internalization is the state we are in when we ignore unhealthy thoughts, stresses, emotions, and actions. We ignore the signs of what is coming while letting semi-unconscious thought patterns push us into damaging activities. We enable an emotional parasite to take over our mind and wreak havoc on our bodies. This process of internalizing and ignoring is a big reason why we fall into harmful behaviours. Even though we understand that the behaviours don't serve our health and lead to both physical and mental anguish, we give them power.

If internalizing and ignoring our stresses, emotions, and unhealthy actions are the problem, what is the solution?

Externalize and investigate

The worst thing you can do when falling into unhealthy patterns is to ignore their emergence. Keeping these thoughts and feelings in our subconscious results in the mindless suffering that happens under the radar of our conscious mind. What we need to do instead is find ways to externalize and investigate these unhealthy thoughts and feelings. I call this objectifying the behaviour. Objectifying your responses, emotions or stresses is the key to taking control of your worst self-harming thoughts and actions. By pushing our thoughts outside ourselves, we can look at them objectively and ask questions about them. We are far less likely to ruminate and lose our power to change damaging mindsets. We have three very distinct opportunities to take advantage of this process before the behaviour takes hold. While this is an unnatural skill that takes lots of practice, if you understand when and how you can use it, you will get better at applying the technique. This vastly increases your chances of success.

The three times we can objectify an unhealthy thought or behavioural pattern are at the moment, after the moment has passed, and before future moments. I call this past, present, and future self-questioning.

Get something out of it

Before we get into the technique of present, past, and future self-questioning, we should touch on the ultimate purpose of this method. Humans are perpetually fallible, and even when we are at our best, we make mistakes. The harm is not in the mistake we make, but rather in the failure to learn from it. When we find ourselves on the wrong end of unhealthy behaviours, we usually get emotional and beat ourselves up over it. When we go down the rabbit hole of uncontrolled unhealthy snacking, we feel guilty, ashamed, and disappointed in ourselves. You are supposed to care about yourself more than anyone else in the world. Still, these internal thoughts are the sad reality of our post behavioural self-talk. What has this sort of negative reflection ever accomplished for you? When has becoming an emotional wreck and increasing your self-hatred ever improved your future decision-making ability or made your life any better? If anything, this sort of self-assault makes your future decision-making markedly worse. You end up respecting yourself less and falling more deeply into unhealthy coping. If you're going to spend the night on the couch instead of going to the gym, you'd better get something out of it. Why not use moments of weakness and lack of control as an opportunity to grow? Present, past, and future self-questioning is all about this idea of getting something out of it.

Step 1: In the Moment

When we are engaged in an unhealthy behaviour, there is always an opportunity to catch ourselves in the act and change the outcome. This isn't easy to do as our programming for harmful behaviour is already strong. Still, with practice, we can get better at nipping the action in the bud. When we are elbow deep in the ice cream tub, we can assess what is happening. Still, we typically avoid facing the reality of our current choice of action. We prefer to mindlessly live within the moment rather than bring the truth of our unhealthy act to the surface. For instance, when you go to the cupboard to grab a few squares of chocolate, you will tell yourself that it is just going to be a small, well-controlled indulgence.

You believe this when you say it to yourself. But what is your mentality when you go back for a second or a third time? When the small indulgence begins to snowball into an entirely different monster, you let the action unconsciously take control of your decision making. You succumb to the idea that this is now out of your control, and it would be less painful to let your craving take hold of the decision-making process. You'll deal with the consequences of your actions at some other time. This is when we find creative ways to either ignore or justify our actions. Your brain is designed to give up long term positive outcomes for short term rewards, even though those short term rewards don't serve your future self. The thing to realize is that at this moment, you have to decide to consciously ignore what is happening. You need to understand that this is a deliberate choice you are making. It may seem like the act of letting something like a craving take hold is unconscious. That is only because your unhealthy programming is so strong. The decision to continue the act of self-harm seems automatic. There *is* an opportunity to make a different deliberate choice. You can choose to ask yourself what is *really* going on and why you are allowing yourself to overeat.

By using the technique of present questioning, you force yourself to investigate the roots of your behaviour and the potential consequences. Here are some examples of questions you can begin to ask yourself when unhealthy behaviours start.

Why am I about to eat this? What is my motivation?

Asking this question forces you to think about what is at hand.

Why are you putting cookies into your mouth in an uncontrolled way?

Are you even hungry? Do you need to eat this snack for some legitimate reason? Did you starve yourself all day long, and has that lead you to crash eating? Is there a healthier option you can switch to instead?

You can no longer successfully lie to yourself about the reality of what is happening once these questions are posed.

How did I feel last time I did something like this?

This line of questioning pushes you to remember the negative consequences of the action. Then you can relate feelings and incidences from memory to the current situation. If you bring the negative emotions that usually come from this action to the surface, there is a good chance that the reminder will push you toward a healthy alternative.

How are you rationalizing or justifying this action?

Just in case you are trying to fool yourself, by using justifications, it can be helpful to ask if you are hiding behind any of them. "I worked hard this week, and I earned this entire large pizza." It is one thing to deny what is happening mindlessly. It is another to continue denying the reality of the situation after you've pointed out the apparent denial to yourself. Think about the stages of denial and where you might be using them to support your current unhealthy state. Quite often, a reality check is all we need to stop the behaviour.

How will you feel about this in 20 minutes, or tomorrow?

Personally, this is my favourite question to ask myself during times of needless indulgence. Is the juice going to be worth the squeeze? These kinds of questions attack our present bias, the tendency to give up future well being for current stimulation. It is helpful to think about the immediate adverse effects of the action you are taking. If you think about the upset stomach and shame you are going to feel after the pizza is gone, you are more likely to assess the action with greater seriousness. If you think about how the action will affect you very shortly, you can often stop it in its tracks.

Is the cost worth this action?

The goal of this question is similar to the prior one. Make yourself admit that the action you are taking is harmful and not worth the pending consequence. What are you trying to get out of this? Stimulation, distraction, numbness? Is the reward worth the physical and mental cost that is going to come once that has ended?

Are you trying to cope with something?

What's going on from an emotional standpoint? You're not hungry. You don't need this food. So why are you eating it? Are you sad? Are you stressed? Perhaps you're bored. What is the motivation here? Is there something you need to surface and deal with that you are burying with food? Is there someone you need to call or an interpersonal issue to resolve? Is there some sort of productive activity that can you can take to heal the roots of your need to cope? Putting energy toward the source of the underlying pain is going to make you feel better. The route of ignoring and self-medicating will only end in future suffering.

Is there a better alternative?

Once you have established that you are aiming to cope with something, can you deal more healthily? Do you need to get out of the house? Could you go for a walk? Is there a friend you can meet? If you don't feel as though you have control over the underlying pain, can you at least find a healthier way to self-medicate?

How will I feel if I don't do this?

This is perhaps the essential "present" question you could ask yourself. How much better will your life be if you don't do what you're doing right now? Will you feel physically better? Will you feel proud of yourself? Will you feel accomplished and in control? Picture what life would be like with and without the unhealthy action. Do you still want to go forward with your current choice after painting a picture of your two potential outcomes?

Summing up present questioning

Present questioning can be very powerful, and the strategy is a clear example of what I mean by "objectifying" your behaviour. When we become aware of the response, put it on the spot, and force ourselves to look at it through the lens of reality, it makes it much more challenging to continue. Objectification of thoughts also allows you to separate yourself from an unhealthy action. You are not your thoughts. You are not even your actions. Emotionally driven comfort-seeking is a symptom of the human condition, not your character. Present questioning is your first line of defence in taking control of your unhealthy thoughts and actions, but it isn't the only line of defence.

Step 2: In the Past

As you can see, present questioning is a powerful tool. It is ideal to be able to nip unhealthy behaviours in the bud when possible. This is what present questioning can accomplish. But, as you and I both know, stopping the action just before it is in full swing isn't always an easy task. Sometimes our first indication of the unhealthy behaviour comes in the form of a belly ache or the regretful and shameful self-reflection that surfaces once the action has stopped. Don't fret. There is a specific line of questioning for this moment as well. While you may not have prevented the unhealthy action, in this case, that doesn't mean you can't get something positive out of the experience. Once the harmful action has already taken place, and you move into the "shame phase," it is the perfect time to use past questioning. This is an intentional form of constructive reflection.

Past questioning is the most abundant opportunity for improvement. Once the action has already happened, the only thing you have left is the opportunity for reflection. Usually, we unconsciously choose to reflect with self-hatred and other defeating attitudes. Still, if you practice, you can look at each slip up as an opportunity to increase your discipline and improve your decision-making ability for the future. Here are some example questions that you can use once the unhealthy action has already taken place.

What's done is done. Now, get something out of it.

Before you investigate your actions, you need to set the landscape for a positive mindset. Without a positive mindset, the rest of the questioning process will cease to be effective. What's done is done. The chips have been eaten. The ice cream is gone. So what is the benefit of beating yourself up over it? We can quickly get sucked into a negative mind-frame after making an unhealthy choice. But it is important to put things into perspective. A single lousy behaviour is going to cause minimal physical damage. It is what the minimal damage does to your mind that can be genuinely harmful. Remember that this is an opportunity to grow and improve. If you allow yourself to adopt a positive outlook, good things can come from seemingly unfortunate events. Don't let the real damage set in. Get something out of it!

What triggered this event? Can you trace it to root habits?

When we find ourselves in the wake of an uncontrolled, unhealthy coping behaviour, we should recognize that it rarely just happens out of the blue. There is a chain of events that led you into the action. Can you trace back to where it began? Have you had an emotional day? Did you have a conflict that usually ends in this type of unhealthy coping? Look back and see if you can find the root of this process. Some people refer to these as "cues." The language is less important than recognizing the precise process. Here's an example:

Behaviour: uncontrolled emotional eating

- Supporting habit 1: I was sitting in front of the T.V. before I turned to food.
- Supporting habit 2: Before I turned on the T.V., I was sitting on the couch, ruminating and quickly becoming bored.
- Supporting habit 3: I was incredibly exhausted after dinner because I had a long, stressful day at work. This is what led me to the couch.
- Supporting habit 4: My day started terribly. I woke up late, rushed out the door, and began my day with the stress of sprinting to work and being disorganized.

- Supporting habit 5: The night before, I was up late, stressing out about the catch up I need to do on a work assignment after months of procrastination. This led to me hitting the snooze button three times and cutting my time short before the day even began.

Root identification: The root of my current uncontrolled eating stems from a procrastination issue. Pushing a project back too late leads to the stress that keeps me from sleeping properly. If I can employ techniques to overcome my procrastination issue, I will solve the root cause of my stress. Thus, I will be able to curb my late-night eating.

This technique may sound complicated, but you could do it in your own life in 5 minutes or less. The more you do it, the more efficient and accurate you become. If you pose the question, the answers will come, and you can identify the causes of your most unhealthy behaviours.

What did the behaviour do for you?

It can be helpful to not only look at the negative aspects of coping but also what the reward was as well. It is not the action that drives us. It is the reward we get as a result of the action. Focusing on the payoff allows you to connect the coping to the pain you are trying to numb. Did the coping relieve boredom? Did it enable you to forget about a stressful situation or a racing mind? Was it pure stimulation you were after? What did the action do for you? Instead of focusing solely on the adverse outcomes of your activities, figure out what the positive effects are, even if the results are positive for a fleeting moment. Once you identify the reward, you can begin to seek out healthier means of achieving the same goal. "The late-night eating took my mind off the fight I had with my parents. The emotional anger I was living with as a result was overwhelmed me. The food distracted me from the pain." When these emotions come up again, try hitting the new punching bag hanging in your basement for 20 minutes or spending time writing down your parents' point of view in an attempt to understand the validity of their actions. This is where readers will want more examples of alternative coping mechanisms, but effective alternatives are highly individual and difficult to recommend. But if you know what the reward of the harmful intervention is, you can seek a healthier option. Play around with it.

Was there a point when you realized you were losing control?

In the present, there are usually a few cues you could have investigated before everything spun out of control. Can you now look back and recall one of these moments? Was there a point where you realized that you were losing control? Could you have asked present questions to slow down and make a better decision? "As soon as I told myself that I'd only have 1 or 2 small cookies, I knew I was lying to myself. I saw a brief flash of my future and the uncontrolled eating that was going to follow. That was my opportunity to get out of the house or get off of the couch. I could have removed myself from the destructive environment."

You don't *have to* create a strategy out of this thinking, although you very well could, and it would be helpful. What's essential in this line of questioning is that you practice becoming more aware of how the behaviour comes into existence and how you allow it to exist.

Was the action worth the outcome?

In reflection, make sure you always note the consequences of your actions. You don't need to do this by beating yourself up. You merely need to observe how the behaviour made you feel at your lowest point. Chances are you will be at a low point when you do this sort of reflection. Note the emotions you are feeling. Are they positive, negative, or neutral? What was the cost of your actions? Was it worth how it has affected you in the present? You don't need to make a plan or have a solution at this moment. You are just training your mind to be more aware, so in the future you can self-regulate in a healthier way.

Always ask what could've been done differently

Could you cope with a less consequential type of food? Could you find relief in physical activity or by performing some breathing exercises or mindfulness techniques? Is there a friend you could've called or met up with to settle yourself down? There is usually a better solution and means of healthy coping you can use instead of your self-harming behaviours. Experiment and find what works for you.

Summing up past questioning

When it comes to past questioning the most important factor is the mindset. If you are negative, defeated, and self-deprecating, it is doubtful that you will create the necessary space needed for proper healing. If you can remember that the damage is done and you have a choice between creating more damage or healing, you are more likely to reflect positively. Just make sure that you put things into perspective and look at every poor choice as an opportunity to make better choices in the future.

Speaking of the future, there is a line of questioning we can follow that can help us make better decisions before engaging in unhealthy behaviours? Future questioning is the line of inquiry we use to create a framework for success in our transformation.

Step 3: For the future

Future questioning is best performed at scheduled times once the emotional repercussions of our most recent adverse event have calmed down. You want to ensure you are in a positive space for self-reflection. Here are some examples of future questioning.

What can I do next time to ensure a more positive outcome?

When we plan for the next personal crisis, we are more likely to ask the right questions when that situation arises. We can create an advantageous mental framework that strengthens both present and past questioning. The more time you spend planning how to handle unhealthy behaviours, the better your chances of preventing them. As soon as you are done suffering your most recent relapse, look back on the incident. Generalize what you could have done at various stages to minimize the consequences.

What do I want for my life, and what actions must I take to accomplish that?

Future forecasting allows you to picture what life would be like if you took better care of yourself and had improved decision-making skills. When you ask yourself what you need to do to create the life you want, you are more likely to be reminded of your values in the future. Ask yourself, "What would my life be like if I started taking control of my health and employing effective brain training strategies right now? What will my life be like in five years if I don't take this seriously, and I slip further into chronic health issues?" Frame what you want and don't want for yourself. This will increase your chances of using effective questioning and mindfulness next time you are heading down a destructive path.

What triggers and emotions make me susceptible to unhealthy behaviours?

This preparatory questioning allows you to note what frame of mind you are usually in when you succumb to your worst behaviours. It will enable you to recognize your negative cues better. Doing so will allow you to catch yourself when you are in a negative headspace, and you will more easily identify what is happening at the moment. If you know that a fight with your mother will turn you angry and resentful, and end with binge drinking, you'll know to avoid that situation in the future. At the least you can work on using mental resilience practices to stabilize this interpersonal experience. Doing either will allow you to mitigate much of the potential damage. Next time your mom sets you off with one of her well-meaning but degrading comments, you can calmly ask present and past questions. Gentle questioning will help put the exchange into perspective. "Mom only says those things because she worries about me and doesn't know how to communicate her feelings better. I don't need to let this be a negative experience." Get yourself in the right headspace for this sort of forgiving conversation by taking 10-20 minutes to do some breathing exercises and "reset" before forming your opinion about the thoughts and feelings of the other side.

Was there a beginning? Could I have seen this coming?

The last thing you can explore when trying to prepare for future self-harming events is finding the root of unhealthy behaviour. We discussed this at length in the previous section. Still, sometimes it can be more useful to implement this process when you are settled. If you know the root of the problem, you can look for it next time. You can even find ways to get rid of it or change it, thus preventing the self-harming behaviour altogether. For instance, if you know late-night snacking begins with sitting on the couch when feeling exhausted after a long day at work, you need to find a strategy to keep you off the couch. Or you need to find a way to find more energy and be less exhausted at night. Perhaps you can do some Yoga in the basement instead, or go into the den and read that book you've wanted to dive into. When it comes to addressing the roots of your worst behaviours, the method is less important than the change in routine that gets you away from going down the same unhealthy path. It is about altering your automatic thoughts and negative core beliefs. If you can slow down the reaction, you can change it. If you can manage the response, you can reduce the need for self-medication. Experiment and make your mind work for you.

Summarizing self-questioning

It takes time for present, past, and future self-questioning to become effective. But like most things, if it works, it takes effort. If you utilize these techniques when you can, you will improve, and over time you'll see greater rewards. You will get to the point where the right questions come to mind automatically. That is what we ultimately want. You are slowing down your system one and giving your system two more significant room to operate and make the right decisions. This sort of brain evolution is what makes you a good decision-maker.

It is best not to have specific expectations about how quickly you will see results from this process. You want a trajectory, but a timeline will only frustrate you. It is much better to keep these questions written down in an accessible place so you can be reminded of them often. List them on your fridge or cupboard, or anywhere that problems are likely to arise. If you are diligent and positive throughout this process, you will be astonished to see just how powerful this objectification of life's worst thoughts, feelings, and actions can be.

Actions dictate your outcomes. Emotions dictate your actions. Train your brain to manage your emotions, and you will achieve your results.

Journaling: A helpful tool

For those who struggle with the present, past, and future lines of self-questioning, I recommend keeping a nightly journal. Journaling can be performed in five minutes or less and is very useful. Each night before going to sleep, pull out a pen and pad of paper and do the steps below.

Write what you want for yourself tomorrow

The first thing you need to write down in the journaling process is what a perfect, healthy day would look like tomorrow. You could write something like, "The perfect day for me would be to wake up feeling refreshed and have a nice, calm breakfast. Breakfast would be followed by a productive, stress-free day at work. This would leave me with enough energy to hit the gym, then spend the evening with a good book and a single glass of wine before going to bed. I could sleep without feeling anxious or overwhelmed." Whatever your version of the "perfect" day is, that's what you want to jot down. It only needs to be a single descriptive paragraph, and you shouldn't spend 20 minutes overthinking the process or re-writing your thoughts in an attempt to perfect them. If the exercise is too demanding, you won't do it.

Write down what it would take to achieve that perfect day

You have your perfect day mapped out. Now, what do you need to do to have the best chance of achieving that ideal day? You'll need to get to bed early enough to get a good sleep. You'll have to have enough time in the morning to relax and have a good breakfast, which also means you need to get to sleep earlier than usual the night before. Maybe you need to consciously lock up your phone and laptop and make a point of getting to sleep right after your journaling is done. At work that day, you'll have to be in control of your emotions and use present questioning to put daily work interactions into perspective and reduce any adverse emotional effects. When you finish work, you'll need to stay motivated enough to go to the gym. Perhaps you should write a post-it reminder on your steering wheel. Try something like, "You may not feel like going to the gym right after work, but once you leave the gym after a great workout, you'll be happy you made an effort."

When you get home and have eaten dinner, you'll be

tempted to jump on the couch and turn on the television. Perhaps you can remind yourself that you wanted to read a book with a glass of wine. T.V. watching leads to less energy and more unhealthy behaviours. Commit to 10 pages of the book, and if you want to read more after that, it's up to you. You'll need to pour your single glass of wine and remind yourself that more than one drink is not joy; it is excess. If you do all of these things to the best of your ability, you shouldn't have any anxiety when you go to sleep. You have actively contributed so much to your well-being today that you will feel accomplished instead. This what it would take to achieve the perfect day.

This, of course, is just an example and may not directly apply to your life, but you get the idea. Saying what you want for yourself out loud and then writing down what you must do to achieve that result will make you more likely to take action going into the next day. You aren't expected to do all of the tasks you set for yourself. So don't set the expectation of consistently achieving a perfect day, at least not at first. As long as you make more positive decisions than you would have otherwise, you are winning the day, and the exercise is doing its job.

Alternative Exercise- The "bad day" example

Some people make better future decisions when thinking about potential negative consequences. Imagining the outcome of a terrible day can be more motivating than imagining the result of a great day. If you're one of these people, follow these steps in place of the previous two.

Write down what your worst day would look like

Just like the "perfect day" scenario, you are going to map

out what the worst scenario for your day could look like tomorrow. Perhaps you wake up late, and this makes you irritable and anxious, resulting in missing breakfast and having to rush out the door in a disorganized mess. You get stuck in traffic on the way into work, and you rapidly become stressed out of your mind. You stop at a drive-thru and stuff your face with a greasy egg and sausage sandwich because it's all you have the time to eat. When you get to work, your boss is all over you about being late. You are already stressed out to the max, and her unhelpful commentary about your delay is not helping matters. You get home and eat comfort food to begin taking the day's pain away. After that, you waddle over to the couch where you spend the next 4 hours going back and forth between the T.V., laptop, wine cabinet, and chip bag until past midnight. You go to bed feeling sick, ashamed, stressed, and disappointed in yourself.

What actions would you have to take to have the worst day?

Just like in the positive scenario, you will follow up on your creation of the "worst day" with the actions you would need to take to make the day a reality. For example, you'd have to go to bed late to wake up exhausted and rushed. You'd have to be unprepared by failing to make a lunch or organizing your breakfast the night before. You'd have to take a specific driving route and go out of your way to hit the fast-food joint and get a greasy "to go" breakfast. We don't need to go through it again, as you can see the point of reverse-engineering the scenario is to demonstrate the potential consequences of negative actions. This can motivate you to implement an affirmative plan or bring your potential harmful pitfalls to the surface. If you are aware of how a bad day begins, you will know what you need to avoid doing to have a great day. Most people will thrive by writing out their perfect day. Still, there is a small segment of people who will find greater success with consequential mental pictures and motivations. Know who you are or play around with both and see what gets you a better result.

Write down how it went

Regardless of whether you choose to go with the perfect day, the worst day, or a version of both in your journaling, the following night, you need to write down how it all went for you. Once you attempted to live the day you journaled about the night before (perfect day) or avoid living the day you journaled about the night before (worst day), you must assess the outcome. What went well, and what strategies from your journaling process were you able to implement successfully? What didn't go well, and what could you have done differently to prevent those negative pieces of your day from coming to life? Don't judge your actions during the process; just investigate them and make sure that you note the positive steps you took as a result of journaling. This step in the process is your way of getting the facts. That way, you know what to repeat and what to cut out of your plan.

Start over

Once you recap how your day went, you must start all over again by picturing the perfect (or worst) day you could have tomorrow. You need to repeat this entire process, day after day after day, until making the right decisions becomes second nature to you.

The process of journaling, acting, and reflecting may seem time-consuming, but it will take 5-10 minutes to complete. Let's be honest; if you're not journaling, you might well be doing something mindless and problematic. Those who claim not to have time for these exercises are *actually* saying, "I don't have confidence in myself." I would suggest that you perform this process every day for a minimum of thirty days. After that, you can decide if you want to keep it up. I journal when I feel my progress starts to slip and feel myself regressing into old habits and negative patterns. At that point, I will spend a week or two journaling until I get back on track. Then I might not need to do it again for another six months. Once you gain a reasonable amount of self-control and discipline, you can do this work as maintenance.

Strategies like the ones discussed in this chapter are by far the most helpful for rebuilding your brain's operating system and improving your behaviour and decision-making ability. Unfortunately, these are also the strategies that people tend to focus on the least. In my estimation, the value of the exercise is not as tangible or familiar as strategies for diet and exercise. It is easy for us to understand how controlling the amount of food we eat equals fewer calories and less weight. When it comes to quantifying how journaling for ten minutes each night equals weight loss, the average person can't make the connection. I encourage you to put more effort into this brain training than you do into your body training. Just give it thirty days and see what happens. In a few months, you will see how effective these strategies can be for your body and mind. Your mental resilience and decision-making patterns are indirectly responsible for the size of your waistline.

Key Takeaways

· *Presence and mindfulness put you in a position to make better decisions. Shake up the circuitry and get off of autopilot with intelligent self-questioning*

· *Be less judgemental. Be interested in what is happening without attaching your negative internal dialogue to every action you take.*

· *Ask questions before, during and after unhealthy behaviours.*

· *In tricky situations, rehearse a mental plan.*

· *Eventually, right-thinking will become the norm.*

When you react, you make bad decisions. When you think, you make better decisions. Unfortunately, you are wired to respond and must train your mind to think more rationally. When you overeat, judge yourself harshly, or become a ball of stress, you are reacting. When you eat the right amount, forgive yourself, and relax, you are accessing your rational mind. Only one type of person can be a successful decision-maker. You know which version of yourself that is.

CHAPTER 9- IN THE EVENT OF A RELAPSE...

"You may have to fight a battle more than once to win it." -- **Margaret Thatcher**

L et me congratulate you on getting to the end of this book. While, in my opinion, much of the material is introductory, I believe it is what you need to understand to see long-term results in your health. If you apply the principles covered in the pages you have read, you will succeed.

A fallacy I see when it comes to succeeding in weight loss is the belief that those who are successful don't make mistakes. On the contrary, those who are successful likely make just as many mistakes as the rest of us. The difference is that the successful person's errors are isolated and dealt with positively. Small mistakes don't prevent successful people from getting right back into an excellent decision-making routine. When an "unhealthy" person makes a poor choice (like stopping at the drive-thru for a cheeseburger because it was the only option on the highway), it can lead to an entire weekend of binge eating and a "forget it" attitude. The mindset becomes distorted and harmful. "I already ruined the weekend, so I might as well just do whatever the hell I want this week." Does this sort of thing sound familiar? The failure mindset is driven by negative self-thoughts like, "You're just not cut out to be healthy.

You should've known all along that this wasn't going to work." The "healthy" person, on the other hand, might slip up at dinner and overeat all the mashed potatoes and get sucked into having a dessert that he didn't need. But the successful person chalks it up to a momentary lapse in judgment that resulted in some stimulation. In the grand scheme of things, it isn't going to affect his health as long as it doesn't snowball into the justification of further unhealthy behaviours. There's no need for restriction or self-punishment to make up for mistakes. Just get back on track and continue with life.

That is the difference between the healthy and the unhealthy mind. It's not about the mistakes you make. It is about how those mistakes determine future behaviour. As I like to say to my coaching clients: a mistake doesn't lead to failure. Two mistakes in a row do.

You are human, and as a human, you are fallible. No matter how badly you want to be perfect, you will have ample opportunity to make poor choices, and you will continue to take many of those opportunities to feel instant gratification at the cost of long term health outcomes. For that reason, it is essential to have a plan in the event of a relapse. This is especially true when it's the kind of regression that has taken hold of your mind and sucked the positivity out of you. Turning around a potential relapse is what this chapter is all about.

Know when you're falling off track

The most critical aspect of preparing for an eventual relapse is recognizing the common signs that the regression is coming. These signs and signals are easy to spot with a well-trained eye or when we are intentionally conscious of them. As with most of our psyche, we are likely to suppress these signals rather than surface and investigate them. Just like how we ignore our emotions, feelings of fullness, and the signs that we are about to fall into an unhealthy behaviour, we ignore what should be obvious. When there are clear signs of falling off track we become afraid. We become fearful of being exactly who the negative voice in our head has always said we are. We become scared of not being powerful enough to take control as we see our progress and hard work slipping away. We are afraid of seeing the relapse coming, doing our best to prevent it from taking hold, and failing anyway. We are protecting our fragile ego that has been cracked and chipped from years of adverse life events. It is natural, but we must nip it in the bud and turn things around before it is too late. So the first thing we need to do is understand that everyone slips up. It isn't just "me."

Everyone has relapses that challenge their resilience and threaten the progress they have made. The concept of "resistance" that Steven Pressfield discusses in his influential book "Do the Work" is an example of this. Steven describes resistance as the voice in our head that is always asking us to give up and take the easy route rather than stick it out and achieve our ultimate potential. Resistance is the unrelenting noise that wants us to remain lifelong failures. This voice never disappears, and the threat of relapse will always exist. Therefore, we require specific tools and strategies to deal with this unrelenting resistance. Understand that when you see the danger of decline on the horizon (or if you find yourself stuck in the midst of one), the first thing you need to do is relax, take a deep breath, and remember that you are in control. The second thing is recognize that no matter how far into a relapse you are, the problem is reversible. The only real damage to your progress occurs if you let the regression take hold of your life and swallow you whole. A series of poor choices must turn into a lifestyle to have a significant effect on your outcome. You need to approach a potential relapse with positivity, forgiveness, and, most importantly, a realistic view. You are not a failure. Your situation is not unique. None of this is about you or who you are as a person. You are a human who is struggling with the barriers discussed in the book. You are designed to fail, but you are powerful enough to overcome these barriers and change your life forever. You must allow power to enter your mind and crowd out the negativity. If you can put things into perspective and be mentally resilient, you will be unstoppable in the face of the most unrelenting relapse.

Examples of recognizing a relapse

Missed Tracking/Logging: If you have implemented diet, exercise, and lifestyle strategies to your life, there is likely going to be some form of progress tracking included. Some people find it helpful to track their food using a small book or one of the many tracking applications available today. Some people do daily or weekly weigh-ins for the sake of accountability or information collection. Some people track their meditation sessions, their active rest, and journaling. Whatever it is you are tracking, you are most likely tracking something. If you aren't, you probably should be. To get the facts and see what you are doing to contribute to your health in an unbiased way, you need some kind of objective information. When we start to have a snowball of unhealthy behaviours that lead to the beginnings of a relapse, we begin to drop out tracking duties. We stop tracking our food, we stop tracking gym visits, and all of the daily work we put into maintaining our transformation plan start to fall by the wayside. We get the attitude of "if things aren't going well, what's the point in writing it down?" The point is that tracking prevents you from escaping the reality of your unhealthy actions. If you let each day pass without objectively documenting the steps you are (or are not) taking to better your health, it is because a part of you has already given up. This can be one of the first and most visible signs of a relapse.

Missed Activities: Let's say for the past few months you've been going to the gym three days per week, doing Yoga once per week, and meditating for 10 mins each morning. In the past few weeks, however, you've been to the gym only once. Perhaps you haven't been to Yoga at all and did just one meditation session. You will tell yourself this is just a "rut" or attribute the lack of action to some other factor, but it is far more likely that you are opening the back door for the eventual escape from your weight loss efforts. When we go from consistent, committed daily actions to more sporadic, casual actions, it is a clear sign that we are mentally checking out. There is a good chance you are letting your discipline slip away and letting "resistance" get the best of you. When you begin to miss regular activities for more then a week, regardless of how you justify it to yourself, you need to be honest and question if there is something else at play. Because the chances are that there is. Just like we know a relationship is losing steam as communication becomes less and less frequent, when the activities that you used to perform become sparse, you are on your way to a relapse.

Slowing of enthusiasm: remember how inspired you were in the first three weeks of January? You were showing up to the gym every day and giving it your all. You even got excited about the thought of exercising. You regularly wrote down your shopping list and looked up new foods and ingredients that you could try out in the kitchen. You bought a bunch of new clothes and exercise equipment to aid you in your transformation. Your enthusiasm was bubbling. Those days are now beginning to feel like they are far behind you. You are looking for excuses to miss the gym, and when you finally drag yourself there, you are more focused on checking your phone than you are on sweating. You secretly hope that the gym has closed due to broken plumbing so that you can stay home. When you go to the grocery store, you buy ready-made foods and spend less time constructively shopping for whole food. You are starting to slip back into your old ways. When you began, you had structure, direction, and enthusiasm, but over time it has started to fade. This is a clear sign that you are mentally checking out and slipping into a full-blown relapse.

Increased excuse-making: The way we frame our poor choices can tell us a lot about where our head is. Let's say you had a pizza last night and ate nine slices. Hey, it's your birthday in 2 weeks, so what's the big deal? Right? Perhaps you missed the gym every day this week. But hey, you had a busy work week. You can't be a gym rat every week. Or maybe you had a little too much social fun last night and woke up hungover this morning. A friend was in town, so why not? That's what you're supposed to do when you haven't seen someone in a while! As we slip into a relapse, we rarely want to admit the harmful nature of our unhealthy behaviours. Where we were once honest and investigative, we become ignorant and suppressive. Increased excuse-making acts as a buffer between our ego and the pending relapse that we are trying to ignore. When excuse-making increases, it is a clear sign that we are trying to protect our ego and ignore the obvious backslide.

Increased doubt and negativity: when negative self-talk increases, we are usually preparing ourselves for failure. Telling ourselves, "You can't do this," and sending other small, doubting internal messages makes the blow less crushing when we quit. If failure is what we expect, who cares if we do fail? When you sense an increase in doubt and negative self-talk, you must recognize it is a defence mechanism that is preventing you from seeing that you are slipping up. You are creating negative framing to avoid a critical ego blow that comes when you give up on yourself. You see this sort of thinking all the time in life. When we want something to happen, we usually voice the lack of potential for a positive result. That way, if the positive effect doesn't come, it was expected. If it does occur, it's a bonus! If you meet a man or woman at a party who you connect with, you might say to yourself, "There's no way he or she is going to call." You desperately want the call to come through, but you're afraid to admit the "want" as wanting leaves you vulnerable. This reverse psychology approach to fear is not your friend, and you must bypass it to see clearly. You must remind yourself of how much you value the goal of taking control of your health. Failure to do so will likely manifest in a relapse.

Those are just examples of common signs of relapse that I see every day. You likely have a few that are unique to you that I didn't note here, so don't limit yourself to this list. The most important takeaway of this section is that there are many visible signs of a future relapse. We can pick up on these signals if we choose to be honest with what our actions are dictating instead of normalizing these red flags to protect our egos. To fail gently is not a wise goal. The thing that all red flags have in common is that they exist as an unhelpful defensive mechanism. Our ego has become fragile from years of adverse life experiences. Our internally produced negative self-images that have come from those adverse events beg for protection. The more expected it is that we will fail, the less vulnerable we become to the hurt when we do. At least that is what we believe. If you allow yourself to be vulnerable enough to dismiss failure as a danger to your ego, you will never get to the point of failure. You will be resilient, prevail in the face of many barriers, and you will persist until you hit your goal. There is only one way to fail, and that is to quit. All other results are just learning experiences that you can use to better your future strategy. Now the question becomes, "How do we prevent the process of relapse once we recognize the sign(s) that one is on the horizon"? Taking action is what we will discuss in the next section.

Normalize the "dips"

The first thing you need to focus on when trying to prevent a recognized relapse is to normalize the scenario in your mind. To slip up is human, and backslides do not equal failure. You're not weak, and slip-ups have nothing to do with who you are as an individual. That is just the story we believe. It is only all part of the process. The question worth asking is, "How are you going to deal with it"? Are you going to ignore the signs that failure is on the horizon and increase your self-doubt? Are you going to succumb to your old ways of thinking and take the back door exit instead of facing the reality that you are veering off your path? To believe that a relapse is coming because something is wrong with you and you are too inadequate to deal with it is the only path to failure. The ball is in your court, and the final decision is always yours. The power lies in you, not in an external circumstance where you can place blame.

Think about using the skills you have developed in your present, past, and future self-questioning to objectify the slip-up and get yourself back to reality. Are you the only person in the world who has fallen off their diet before? Do a few weeks of poor choices undo all of the efforts you put into the months beforehand? Is it outside of your power to take back control and go back to your healthy routine? The answer to all of these questions is, of course, "no," but if you don't pose them to yourself in an objective way, you will allow your defensive thinking to cannibalize your mind. You can't think within the lines of reality while letting your harmful, automatic thoughts run rampant. When you see the signs of a relapse, you need to gather yourself, put things into perspective, and get back on track. There isn't any rush to add one hundred healthy habits back into your life in that second, but you need to get your mind right and put one foot in front of the other. Just begin to shift back into your healthy routine one step at a time. Remember that recovery starts with the realization that this sort of thing happens, and it is O.K. Success is as simple as getting back into a routine of healthy choices, one choice at a time.

Find Positivity in the Failure

The easiest way to stop relapse in its tracks is by finding positivity in your perceived failure. This can be difficult to do, but if you've spent some time using self-questioning to "get something out of" minor daily behavioural slip-ups, you will be prepared to utilize this thinking when you need it. If you haven't used the method of self-questioning to build this skill of resiliency and objectification, now is a great time to start.

The first thing you should remind yourself of when recognizing a relapse is the value of feeling low. You don't feel great about yourself right now, and the unhealthy choices you've allowed to pile up over the last few weeks did not deliver on their subconscious promises of comfort and safety. When you decided to stop exercising and give up on your healthy eating in exchange for T.V., chips, and your smartphone, it didn't work out. At the time, you might've received some much welcomed numbing and distraction through food and laziness, but how is that working out now? It can help to remind yourself of what your motivation was for unhealthy actions, and what the contrasting result ended up being. The indulgences haven't delivered. If you want to feel good about yourself again and improve, you just need to go back to healthy actions.

Look at your slip-up as nothing more than a temporary psychological break from dieting. When you make significant changes to your diet and exercise routine, you get a rate of diminishing returns, both physiologically and psychologically. For example, once you lose around 10% of your starting weight, your body begins to slow your metabolism and bring down your enthusiasm for exercise to increase your energy (caloric) surplus. Your body does this because it does not want you to lose weight. Your body can also bring down your mental strength and increase your psychological cravings for the very same reason. Because of this, it is sometimes beneficial to step away from your diet and exercise interventions and let yourself "reset." Of course, this isn't exactly what happens when you unintentionally go on a binge. But that doesn't mean you can't turn it into something positive. The "reset" mentality should be executed intentionally, but if you get there unintentionally, just look on the bright side. You slipped up for a bit, and perhaps your mind and body needed it, but now the actions aren't serving you anymore. You feel awful about yourself both physically and mentally, so it's time to regroup and move back into health mode.

There is always something you can get out of a temporary slip up if you choose to guide your mind in the direction of positivity, and at the end of the day, you'll only be stronger for it. Look at your slip up as an opportunity to rise to the occasion and change your negative cycle of thinking. You can be stronger after a relapse if you want to be, so choose a positive mindset and receive a positive outcome.

Go back to the basics

Once you have addressed your mindset and gotten over the idea that your transformation has to end over a few "bad days", it is time to go into recovery mode. The worst thing you can do right now is try to make up for your unhealthy behaviours through extreme counteractions. If you come back to your weight loss routine with more restriction, increasingly intense activity, and more obsession about your routine, you might be setting yourself up for disaster. There is a good chance you tried to do too much too fast in the first place, which is partially responsible for what leads you into a relapse. There's an even better chance that throwing too much change into the mix when you're still a little "fragile" from the collapse is going to end up overwhelming you and increasing your emotional frustrations. If you are already emotionally "down," substantial caloric restriction and increased exercise intensity can only add to your potentially overflowing stress bucket. It could even become an eating pathology. If you have a flat tire, it is best not to push the gas pedal to the floor to resolve being stuck. It's better to take your time, patch the hole, and slow down on the highway until you can get a new tire on the car. The same principle applies here. You want to go back to the very basics of lifestyle change. Think about the two to three actions you can add back into your daily routine that are going to make the most significant impact on your health, preferably with the least amount of effort. For instance, if you have slipped back into the habit of going to bed very late, snacking all night long, and then eating at the drive-thru because you are rushing out the door, there isn't much point in planning to go to the gym seven days per week. The first thing you need to do is get into bed before 10 PM. Perhaps you can add in an evening habit like stretching, walking, or reading to get you away from the couch and the television. These sorts of minor, doable changes are going to be much more effective and impactful than running on the treadmill for two hours each day on an empty stomach in an attempt to burn away calories that stem from your guilt. Don't rush your way back to making "progress," primarily through actions that are not the source of your setbacks. Get back to the most basic self-care routine that will allow you to recover from a psychological perspective before you worry about the physiological outcome.

Here are a few ideas of habits you can try to integrate back into your lifestyle instead of punishing yourself back to "health" with restriction and exercise obsession.

- Go back to late-night journaling

- Spend 10-20 mins each morning or evening working on stretching and breathing exercises

- Make your breakfast and dinner every day (or when you can)
- Don't eat out for the entire week

- Do something active (but not intense or prolonged in duration) each day

- Limit your T.V. time to one show per night

- Get to bed by 10 PM each weekday

You get the idea. Focus on long-term habits and routines that set you up to succeed in your diet and exercise efforts first. Then you can go back to making diet and exercise efforts. Small habits support more substantial behavioural changes, and the magnitude of your habits is less critical than their repeatability. It doesn't work in reverse. If you want to get back to seeing results from your diet and exercise efforts, you must first create the habit and behavioural patterns that stick more easily.

Aim to reintroduce one new habit per week or every two weeks, and track your daily adherence to that action. You can do this with a notepad, a smartphone, or an excel spreadsheet. Just write down the habit you are currently trying to mix back into your routine with a seven-day box, and at the end of each day, tick the box if you completed the habit. If you don't hit 90% adherence after two weeks, don't add another habit. Keep doing this until you are back into a routine. Making a comeback will leave you stronger and more confident! If you can recover once, you can do it every time it happens in the future, and that is the key to sustainable, long-term change. The ability to make a comeback is a powerful psychological weapon.

Don't change too much too quickly

As you go through the schedule of slowly adding back high impact habits, don't get ahead of yourself. If your first habit reintroduction is to go for a 30-minute walk each evening when you would typically sit on the couch, don't try to turn a 30-minute walk into a 2-hour walk after the first day. Stick to maintaining the small, doable goal for at least a few weeks, then reassess. If you commit to getting back to the gym three days per week, don't decide that you are going to do back to back classes on your second day. Just stick to the plan. Implementing too many habits at one time can do more harm than good, and so can the act of increasing complexity and intensity within those scheduled reintroductions. It is excellent that you are inspired and motivated again. Still, over-exercising and under-eating based solutions stem from the most cynical sources of motivation and should be avoided at all costs. You want to conserve enough energy to continue implementing a new habit every one to two weeks. If you try to increase the frequency, intensity, or complexity of the reintroduced practices too quickly, you will overload yourself and fall back into another relapse. The most challenging thing for a person is patience, but lack of patience has never gotten you anywhere in the past, so keep that reality in mind while trying to pull back the reins on your habit reintroductions. Slow and steady wins the race. That isn't just a fable. It is true to life.

As time passes, focus on synergy

A few months have gone by, and you've successfully made a few new habit introductions. Things are going great. Your weight is down, your self-talk is positive, and you feel terrific. Now it is time to focus on the synergy of the habits you are reintroducing. As you continue to add patterns into your routine, you will want to begin integrating new practices from different areas of lifestyle to create the necessary synergy for success. You don't want to start adding back only dietary habits, or only exercise habits, or only sleep and stress management habits. Once you have added back your 2-3 high impact, doable practices with success, I advise you to start spreading them around. You will want to reintroduce a food habit, then an exercise habit, then a sleep habit, then a stress management habit, then an active rest and recovery habit. Start adding a different category of practice each week that can integrate with the patterns that you introduced before it. The order does not matter nearly as much as the variance within the category of the reintroduction. Exercise feeds sleep and stress management, and a well-slept person makes better nutritional decisions. That is one example of why synergy matters when it comes to building back your routine. Below is an example to show you exactly what I mean.

Week 1-2: Make my dinner from scratch every day
Week 2-4: Go for a walk for 30-60 minutes after dinner each night
Week 4-6: Journal my "perfect day" before bed
Week 6-8: Do 10 minutes of meditation before my journaling
Week 8-10: Write down my past and future thinking for the day before dinner
Week 10-12: Start preparing my lunch at night for the next day
Week 12-14: Swim at the aquatic centre every Sunday

Some people would refer to this as a form of "habit stacking." When you get back into the groove of reintroducing your healthy habits, make sure the approach becomes a well rounded one. Each different contribution improves your likelihood of adherence to all of the others. Stress management is going to improve your sleep. More energy is going to lead to more exercise. More exercise is going to reduce the likelihood of spending all night on the couch. Staying off the sofa is going to reduce your harmful eating patterns. That's synergy. As you reintroduce new habits week after week to regain traction, make sure to mix it up to get the best results.

Summary

When you start to slip and fall into a pending relapse, you must:

1. Recognize the common signs and bring the reality of the relapse to the surface.

2. Relax, be rational, and approach the regression with positivity. This can be an opportunity.

3. Go back to basics once you have mentally recovered.

4. Introduce new habits every 7-14 days and don't move on until 90% adherence is hit.

5. Increase the synergy of your reintroductions once the ball is rolling, by adding habits from a variety of different areas of lifestyle.

As I mentioned earlier, this is an opportunity. It isn't just some cheesy mindset strategy. This is your chance to break the cycle of failure that has haunted you in the past. This is your opportunity to test yourself and prove that the work you have put in is paying off. It is a pivotal event in your journey where you can look back and say, "that was the moment it all changed. That was the moment that *I* changed." And this event is inevitable, so prepare for it. You have it within you to achieve a positive outcome under the direst circumstances. You just need to put yourself in the proper frame of mind to see failure for what it is: a bump in the road that we allow to grow due to ego-driven fear. Whether it remains a bump that you gently drive over or it develops into a wall that you could never scale is really up to you. I know the thought of having that kind of power is scary, but it's frightening because you've never had the mindset to exercise it and believe in yourself. Make this moment different from all the others, and you will never be the same person or suffer the same fate again.

Key Takeaways

· *Good things don't last forever. Don't be shocked when the scale goes the other way. Just remember that you are always one decision away from taking back the controls*

· *The more success you see, the more declines you will have. You need to become less sensitive to relapses if you are going to succeed in the long run*

· *Regression can be a bump in the road or a brick wall. Your attitude determines the size of the hurdles you face.*

· *Failure only exists when you refuse to get back on the horse.*

I often gain 15 - 20 pounds at some time of the year. When that happens, I simply change my behaviour and lose weight. I'm not trying to sound like a jerk when I say that. It's just literally how it happens. I am non-emotional, without fear, and I don't attach the weight gain to who I am as a person. If I did, I would not be a healthy version of myself. I would be too defeated to turn around a regression. You need to be prepared for your decline because it is coming. Life does not move in a continuous, linear slope. Just remember that this is true for both upward and downward trajectories. When things aren't going well, it is only a matter of time until they are. That is assuming you take the right actions and refuse to let a relapse defeat you.

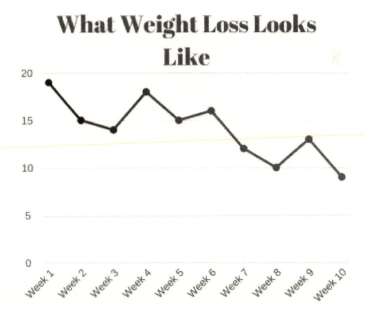

What Weight Loss Looks Like

*weightloss, and progress of any kind, is not a linear process. You must be able to ride the wave and stay positive when it looks like you are struggling. Taking a long view and measuring your progress over months and years is a better approach than the short view.

CLOSING THOUGHTS

This is the end of our time together, but chances are, your journey is just beginning. If you had the determination to make it through the book without the need to be baited by "diet and exercise" magic, you are very likely to begin a process of long term, sustainable health change. You're already well on your way.

I want to tell you what I hope for you moving forward. First, I hope that you understand that the underlying issues and barriers that got you to a poor state of health have very little to do with your personality or character. The evolutionary factors that you don't have any control over are the real culprits. Your insatiable cravings, your uncontrolled snacking, your tendency to overeat, your default toward laziness, and even your highly efficient ability to store body fat are all by design. Knowing this, I hope you stop blaming your worst health behaviours on who you are as a person. Weight gain doesn't stem from internal weakness.

My next hope for you is that you'll understand that while the existence of your health issues is not your fault, turning them around is your responsibility. Now that you have an understanding of where these issues stem from and what you can do to take control of them, the ball is in your court. Your excuses are now invalid, and from this point forward, you have nobody else to blame for your state of health, so take ownership. Nobody is coming to save you. This frame of mind can be empowering as it puts the control back into your hands. If you can overcome your fear and ego, life will get easier and more enjoyable.

My third hope for you is that you come to terms with the fact that taking control of your health is not a short term game. If you aren't in this thing for the long haul and willing to commit at least one year of your life to a process, your chances of success are slim. If, however, you understand that failure only exists in your mind and can only manifest if you quit, all other relapses become an opportunity to learn and grow.

My fourth hope for you is that you move away from diet and exercise centricity and focus on the process of addressing the underlying causes of your most unhealthy habits and behaviours. Please learn more about yourself and the root causes that drive you to self-medication and self-harming acts. I want to see you put as much effort into lifestyle factors like sleep quality, stress management, and becoming a genuinely active person as you have put into your diet and exercise efforts in the past. Lifestyle factors will determine your ability to adhere to your diet and exercise efforts in the long term. As you now know, this is the key to success in your health.

My final hope for you is that you never look for another quick fix. If I have done my job and connected with you, you will no longer be tempted by the trends, fads, and gurus. I want you to see through the promise of a lighter body at the cost of a lighter wallet. I hope this is the only book you will ever need to create your success rather than always looking for external sources to rescue you from your worst habits and outcomes. You are strong, and you are powerful. You are all you need, and I sincerely hope you can begin to believe that truth.

So as we say goodbye to one another, I would like to thank you for reading this book and putting your faith in my ideas. I know that is a difficult thing to do when others have failed you. It has been a sincere pleasure sharing everything I have learned in my professional career and letting go of it so others can have open access. These are my most powerful thoughts and advice. Now they are yours, too. I sincerely thank you for seeing the value of this book. It says a lot about where you are in your journey and how ready you are to take control of your health.

Now go and get what is yours.

ABOUT THE AUTHOR

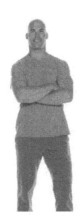

Tommy Caldwell is a behavioural change coach and fitness expert who works out of Hybrid Fitness in London, Ontario. Tommy founded Hybrid Fitness in 2009, and since then, he has worked with thousands of clients, including some of the world's top athletes. Tommy holds designations in Sports Nutrition and Sport Psychology, Counselling, and Cognitive Behavioural Therapy. He also holds his Masters in Business. Tommy continues to reside in London, Ontario, with his wife and three young children. You can find Tommy's work at www.tommycaldwell.net

Manufactured by Amazon.ca
Bolton, ON

17339975R00132